INTERNATIONAL REVIEWS OF THE FAT 2 FIT PROGRAM

Russ and Jeff are regular guys that have been there and done it. They explain it in plain language and make it easy to understand.

—*American iTunes Review*

... an awesome job giving relevant, motivational and often scientifically-backed advice about losing weight the sensible way.

—*Australian iTunes Review*

This is for everybody who would like to lose weight and keep it off.

—*German iTunes Review*

These guys really know what they are talking about—what's more they talk from experience so you know it is real-world advice. Brilliant!

—*U.K. iTunes Review*

Russ and Jeff have this stuff figured out and they present it well. In an industry filled with BS, they cut right through it and offer sage advice, motivation, and the kind of even keel needed on a long worthwhile journey towards health, fitness and overall good karma, and these guys have got that.

—*Canadian iTunes Review*

The F2F plan is the most realistic, sustainable, and sensible plan that I have ever come across in my many years of "dieting." Jeff and Russ explain all the science behind the Fat 2 Fit methodology.

—*American iTunes Review*

Their approach to their audience is tempered by compassion from traveling the same road.
—*American iTunes Review*

... plenty of well-researched information on how to lose weight and get fit—painlessly!
—*U.K. iTunes Review*

No hype, no gimmicks, no junk, no products being promoted, no short-term diet plans, and most importantly NO BULL.
—*American iTunes Review*

If you want to lose weight and keep it off, and get fit without ever really feeling you have to run a marathon every day—this is for you.
—*U.K. iTunes Review*

Kind of a "Myth Busters," but for fitness!
—*American iTunes Review*

...so much no-nonsense info that works! No quick fixes here, but a slow and steady journey to lifelong health and weight maintenance.
—*Canadian iTunes Review*

They are never afraid to tell you like it is, and really help filter through all the "diet and fitness" noise out there.
—*American iTunes Review*

... such a positive and empowering resource for me as I've been dramatically changing my lifestyle this year.
—*American iTunes Review*

You've changed my life and my gratitude is off the charts!
—*American iTunes Review*

I'd be lost without this sound advice.
—*American iTunes Review*

FAT 2 FIT

GETTING THERE & STAYING THERE

from the creators of FAT 2 FIT RADIO
JEFF AINSLIE & RUSS TURLEY

Disclaimer The information and recommendations in this book are for educational and informative purposes only and are not intended as medical or professional advice. Any application of the recommendations set forth in this book is at the reader's discretion and sole risk. All people should consult a doctor before starting any diet or exercise program. The ideas, procedures and suggestions are not to be considered as a substitute for consulting with your physician for any health related matter. While every effort has been made to ensure the accuracy of any internet addresses at the time of publication, neither the publisher or the authors are responsible for changes that occur after the date of publication. Third-party websites are not under the control of the publisher or authors.

*A special thanks to the following people, without whom
this book would not have been completed:*

*The listeners of Fat 2 Fit Radio for sending in their questions, tips, suggestions
and the stories of their weight loss journeys. You made each show more
interesting, educational and inspiring.*

Jacqueline Ainslie for her help in editing this book.

*Giselle Weyte for the hard work in the design and layout of this book. See more
of her work at www.giselleweyte.com.*

CONTENTS

NUTRITION: THE FIRST PILLAR OF LIFE-LONG SUCCESSFUL FAT LOSS

EXERCISE: THE SECOND PILLAR OF LIFE-LONG SUCCESSFUL FAT LOSS

MOTIVATION: THE THIRD PILLAR OF LIFE-LONG SUCCESSFUL FAT LOSS

THE CHALLENGES OF WEIGHT LOSS

WEIGHT LOSS IN THE REAL WORLD

INTRODUCTION

THIS BOOK IS THE CULMINATION of the weight loss topics covered in the first 100 episodes of Fat 2 Fit Radio.

Fat 2 Fit Radio began in 2007 and over the course of three years spread to many countries around the world. The first 100 episodes of Fat 2 Fit Radio were designed to be motivational and educational. The main focus of the show has been to cut through all of the weight loss hype and provide a weight loss plan that works for everybody and works in the long term. The progression of topics were designed to give the listeners all of the tools that they would ever need for lifelong weight loss success.

In each episode, a specific health or weight loss related topic was covered in detail and several listener questions were answered. After several dozen shows, one of the most common listener requests was for a specific show number for a previous topic or question. When listeners wanted a refresher about negative-calorie foods or advanced weight loss techniques for example, they didn't want to listen through dozens of hours of archived shows to find it. As well, new listeners felt that they needed to listen to 50 or 60 hours of programming to get caught up.

This book was written as a response to this so there would be one central archive for our entire weight loss body of work. Listeners to the show can use this book as a quick reference, and people who have not had the opportunity to listen to the show can read everything that they have missed.

It is a logical progression starting with the philosophy of how to achieve success in weight loss, to the finer details in nutrition and exercise, and finally, how to put it all together in the real world.

Fat 2 Fit Radio is the second incarnation of The Fat Guy Radio Show started by Russ Turley. During these broadcasts, listeners followed Russ as he dieted and lost 60 pounds. Like most people, when the diet ended, the weight came back on. Jeff Ainslie reached out to Russ in the effort to help Russ lose his weight for the very last time. They joined forces to create Fat 2 Fit Radio which focused on permanent weight loss and lifestyle changes and followed Russ as he lost almost 100 pounds and kept it off.

THE FAT 2 FIT PHILOSOPHY FOR PERMANENT FAT LOSS

Chapter 1

"Obstacles are the things we see when we take our eyes off our goals."
—*Zig Ziglar*

OUR FAT LOSS PHILOSOPHY

OUR PHILOSOPHY IS NOT TYPICAL of any other diet program today. We do not care how much you will weigh in five days, two weeks or even a month from now. Your body fat level one, five or even 10 years from now determines the success of a fat loss program. Our philosophy is based upon and modeled after the successful strategies and techniques of people who have lost considerable amounts of body fat, and have never gained it back. Here are the six pillars of our philosophy:

1 Diets don't work.

New York Times' most popular diet books, with their diverse range of diets and weight loss programs, do not work. Commercial diet centers which provide pre-packaged foods do not work. Weight loss support groups and networks do not work.

All diet programs work in the short term while people are follow them, but almost all fail in the long run. When a person goes off of a diet or leaves a support network, their body quickly returns to its previous shape.

2 If you want to be a thinner and healthier person, live the lifestyle of a thinner and healthier person.

If you start living the lifestyle of that thinner person right now, rather than when you reach your goal weight, you will never have to go off of any temporary diet.

Look at an active, healthy person who has broken their leg. If they are forced to be sedentary for a couple of months, they will probably gain some body fat. When they get mobile again, the weight comes right off. They don't go on any sort of diet, they just start eating and exercising like the thinner healthier person that they were and still are, and their body catches up again. Live as if you are that thinner healthier person now, and your body will catch up too.

3 Undereating will lead to overeating.

Your body is designed to survive. You can starve yourself in the short term, but your body's desire to live will always win. Willpower can work for a few days or weeks, but it will be no match for the intense food cravings from your body.

4 For long term weight loss, you must go slow.

If it took five years to put on the weight, don't expect to take it off in five months. Rapid weight loss causes you to lose more than just fat. Rapid weight loss can damage your metabolism and cause muscle loss, which will make it easier to gain fat in the future. The goal should be fat loss—not just weight loss.

5 Live the lifestyle of health—not perfection 100% of the time.

You do not have to be perfect to attain a healthy, strong and lean body. If you constantly deny yourself your favorite sinful foods, you will only crave them more. There is no need to feel guilt over a meal like Thanksgiving, Christmas or even a wedding reception.

Healthy, active people enjoy food and events once in a while; chronic dieters lose their ability to enjoy these things.

It is not important what you eat between Christmas and New Year's; what is important is what you eat between New Year's and Christmas.

6 Goal setting is important for success.

Goal setting is the key to get results in the short term, and to keep yourself on track for the long term. How do you know if you have arrived, if you don't know where you were trying to go?

SIMPLY PUT, IF YOU FAIL TO PLAN, YOU PLAN TO FAIL.

Chapter 2

"The difference between try and triumph is just a little umph!"
—Marvin Phillips

EAT MORE, WEIGH LESS

D O YOU WANT TO BE able to eat the most amount of great-tasting food that you can, and still be a thin and fit person? Of course you do! Who wants to live by only eating lettuce for the rest of your life?

You don't have to be constantly hungry to get to your goal weight or to maintain your goal weight. It is possible to reach your goals and maintain them without being hungry. In fact, this is the key for long term success.

Most diet plans advertise the speed of weight loss as one of their advantages. Unfortunately, these diet plans set people up for failure in the long run and guarantee repeat business.

Our goal on Fat 2 Fit Radio has never been speed of weight loss—our goal is permanent weight loss. Since the start of the show, Russ has been slowly losing weight and reporting his weight loss on each show. Over the last few years, he has averaged a little less than one pound of weight loss per week. In the last two years, his weight has plateaued, but he has never gained back weight. At the time of this writing, he is approaching his goal of a 100-pound weight loss.

In the past, Russ has a 100% success rate at being able to lose weight, and a 100% failure rate at gaining the weight back after he stops "dieting." This is also true for close to 100% of our listeners.

We have many listeners who have contacted the show to tell us how fast they are losing weight. At the same time, many also let us know that in their opinion, Russ wasn't losing weight fast enough. At the time, Russ was only losing two or three pounds a month and most of these people were losing somewhere around 10 pounds a month.

Several of these people contacted the show a year or two later to let us know that they were starting over their weight loss programs again.

Now Russ was 40 or 50 pounds ahead of them. He didn't go through months and months of starving and then the inevitable weight gain after. Slow and steady does win the race in the end. You are not going to "diet" intensely, get to your goal weight and then never worry about eating again for the rest of your life. You just have to start eating for the rest of your life right now.

Under-eating will always lead to overeating. What we suggest to do is figure out the number of calories that you will be able to eat to maintain your goal weight, and then just start eating those calories right now and for the rest of your life. If you can handle eating the proper number of calories right now without being hungry, you will be able to get to—and more importantly, maintain—your goal weight for the rest of your life.

This concept is so simple, yet many people have a very hard time believing that it could possibly work. In show #83, we answered an email from a woman who was 5′5″ and weighed 245 pounds. She was eating between 1200 and 1350 calories per day in an attempt to lose weight. Her doctor told her that she was starving herself, every index she referred to told her she wasn't eating enough, and our show was also telling her to eat more. She simply didn't believe that it would be possible for her to eat any more food.

We estimated that if she was a fairly sedentary person, to maintain her weight at 245 pounds, she would need to eat about 2600 calories per day. If she ate that much every day, her weight would stay around 245 pounds. If she lost 100 pounds and now weighed 145, she would be able to eat about 2000 calories per day to maintain that new weight. In this example, a person who weighs 245 pounds only eats an average of 600 calories per day more than a person who weighs 145.

If she changes her lifestyle right now to that of a 145-pound person, she can eat 2000 calories right now. By continuing to eat 2000 calories per day, she will eventually get to 145 pounds and maintain that weight in the long term. When someone says that they don't think they can live the lifestyle of a thinner person, that is simply not true.

This might be shocking, but when she was eating 1200 calories per day, that is the lifestyle of someone who weighs under 50 pounds! She was trying to eat like a five-year-old. Who wants to live like that?

This is a very important topic. The belief that you have to starve yourself to become a thin and healthy person, is probably one of the biggest reasons that people can't seem to lose and keep the weight off. Undereating will always lead to overeating. You cannot fight your body's natural desire to survive. Nobody has enough willpower to keep starving themselves.

The average 140-pound woman eats about 2200 calories to maintain her weight. The average 175-pound man needs to eat about 2500 calories. The average commercial diet for a woman is around 1200 calories, and for a man is around 1500 calories. When a person goes off a starvation diet, they have slowed down their metabolism and increased their cravings. This is a certain recipe for rebound weight gain.

Nobody wants to be hungry for years at a time with only temporary results.

Nobody wants to be hungry for years at a time with only temporary results. Nobody wants to be starving themselves and not seeing results. Think of your five-year goal. Do you want to lose 150 pounds in total with many diets over those five years and still be overweight, or do you want to lose those extra 35 pounds once, over a year, and be living as a slender person for the last four of those years?

Chapter 3

"In order to succeed, your desire for success should be greater than your fear of failure." —Bill Cosby

YOUR BASAL METABOLIC RATE (BMR)

THIS IS ONE OF THE most important concepts in this entire book. Confusion over the Basal Metabolic Rate accounts for the majority of all dieting problems and rebound weight gain.

A human body can be thought of as a car. People and cars both need fuel for energy to move. The more a person moves, the more fuel they use.

Eventually a car has to stop at a red light and while it is waiting, its engine idles. Power is available for the radio and headlights, the air conditioning is running, and the drive train is just waiting for the accelerator to be pressed. Unless it is shut off, it's always burning fuel. Your body works exactly the same way.

A person's engine never turns off during life. When a person is asleep, or even in a coma, their engine is always running. Energy is used for all of the metabolic processes that keep us alive. A person's heart pumps blood, the muscles in the diaphragm and ribs allow us to breathe, even our air conditioning in the form of our sweat glands are active.

The minimum amount of energy that is required to keep a person alive is known as their Basal Metabolic Rate (BMR).

If a person is in a coma and has no voluntary movement, they will burn calories at their BMR. That person can survive as long as they receive their BMR level of calories. If that person is fed less, they will eventually die of starvation.

A person's body knows if it is starving to death. If a person is eating below their BMR level, their body will quickly sound an alarm and start preparing itself for a famine. It will do whatever it takes to stay alive. The first thing it will do is try to slow down its metabolism and reduce the number of calories that it needs each day to survive. Muscle burns a lot of calories, so it will start to digest and destroy muscle tissue to slow down its BMR.

The immediate survival response when eating below the BMR level is not only to burn fat, it is also to reduce your muscle mass to lower the body's metabolism.

The shocking truth of most diets is that they recommend that you eat below your body's Basal Metabolic Rate. This causes severe stress to the body, and once the survival response kicks in, it leads to weight loss plateaus and severe food cravings.

Here is how you can calculate your BMR on paper:

Women   BMR = 655 + (4.35 x weight in pounds) + (4.7 x height in inches) − (4.7 x age in years)

Men   BMR = 66 + (6.23 x weight in pounds) + (12.7 x height in inches) − (6.8 x age in years)

Fat 2 Fit Radio also has a calculator online at www.fat2fitradio.com. Click on "Tools" at the top right, and then choose "Calories and Basal Metabolic Rate."

Here is a table that will provide some examples of BMR results:

SEX	AGE	HEIGHT	WEIGHT	BMR
Male	30	5'9"	185	1900
Male	30	6'2"	250	2350
Female	30	5'6"	150	1475
Female	30	5'10"	200	1700

The results in this table are surprising for most people. Many people think that a diet should only have 1000 or 1200 calories per day. At those levels, almost everyone would be eating below his or her BMR, a recipe for weight loss failure.

Should people eat at their current Basal Metabolic Rate? No, you should not eat at your body's minimal survival level. The minimum level of calories to safely eat per day would be 20% higher than your BMR.

If your BMR is 1900 calories, your minimum daily caloric intake would be 2280 while losing fat (1900 x 1.2) If your BMR is 1500 calories, your minimum daily caloric intake would be 1800 while losing fat (1500 x 1.2).

Is this the amount of calories I should eat per day to lose weight? Not quite, this is the minimum guideline. The next chapter will tell you the exact number.

Chapter 4

*"If my mind can conceive it, and my heart can believe it,
I know I can achieve it."* —*Jesse Jackson*

YOUR SPECIFIC CALORIE LEVEL

A PERSON'S BASAL METABOLIC RATE (BMR) is similar to the amount of energy that a car uses when it is idling at a red light. When that car starts driving, it burns fuel at a much faster rate. Just like a car, all of the activities that a person does throughout the day will increase its energy needs. Going to work, cleaning house, walking, and even chewing gum burns calories over and beyond a person's BMR. How do you determine how many calories each and every single activity burns that you do throughout the day?

Introducing the Activity Multiplier
The Basal Metabolic Rate is the starting point. To determine an approximation of your daily caloric needs, multiply the BMR by the appropriate activity ratio. This result will be the average number of calories that can be consumed to maintain a person's current weight.

Multiply Your BMR by the Appropriate Activity Ratio

- If you get little or no exercise, multiply your BMR by 1.2.
- If you exercise lightly or take part in easy sports one to three times a week, multiply your BMR by 1.375.
- If you are moderately active (three to five times a week) multiply your BMR by 1.55.
- If you are very active (hard exercise or sports six to seven times a week) multiply your BMR by 1.725.
- If you are extra active (very hard exercise or sports and a physical job) multiply your BMR by 1.9.

The following table will illustrate this concept for a person who has a Basal Metabolic Rate of 1500 calories.

PERSON WITH BASAL METABOLIC RATE OF 1500 CALORIES		
LIFESTYLE	**ACTIVITY**	**CALORIES TO MAINTAIN CURRENT WEIGHT**
Couch potato, no exercise	1.2	1800
Office worker, occasional sports or trips to a fitness facility	1.375	2050
Dedicated exerciser on most days of the week, with cardio & resistance training.	1.55	2325
Competitive athlete, training most days of the week & playing competitive sports	1.725	2600
Competitive athlete at night & physical job during the day such as a construction worker or lumberjack	1.9	2850

This table clearly shows that the more activity you do, the more food that you can eat on a daily basis to maintain your weight.

An interesting activity would be to calculate your current daily caloric needs right now, and then also calculate what your needs would be at your goal weight. You may be surprised how close they really are.

Here are two examples:

> **5′5″ woman, 30 years old who exercises lightly (BMR x 1.375)**
> 175 pounds – 2165 calories per day
> 125 pounds – 1850 calories per day
> *The difference is only 315 calories!*

If this 175-pound woman continued to eat 1850 calories per day and exercised lightly, she would eventually become that 125-pound woman.

> **5′10″ man, 30 years old who exercises lightly (BMR x 1.375)**
> 225 pounds – 2950 calories per day
> 175 pounds – 2550 calories per day
> *The difference is only 400 calories!*

If this 225-pound man continued to eat 2550 calories per day and exercised lightly, he would eventually become that 175-pound man.

Chapter 5

"Instead of thinking about where you are, think about where you want to be. It takes twenty years of hard work to become an overnight success." —*Dale E. Turner*

GOAL SETTING

GOAL SETTING WILL TRULY DETERMINE if you will succeed in your weight loss and fitness goals—it is really that simple. Even if you know everything about health and fitness, that will not get you in shape, lower your body fat percentage, improve your cardiovascular fitness or make you one iota healthier.

The saying "knowledge is power" isn't exactly right. Knowledge is only potential power. You must also be motivated to put into practice all of your knowledge. Not just for one or two days, you have to figure out how to keep yourself motivated for the long term.

The Basics of Goal Setting

If you don't plan, you plan to fail. People of greatness don't just happen to do great things by accident. You just can't hope to stumble aimlessly through life and achieve great things.

Goals must be measurable. If you can't measure it, you can't improve it. How would you know that you are on track without being able to measure your results? For example, don't just say that you are going to eat a little less, be specific.

You must set small goals that are easily attainable. If your goal is to do a journey of 1000 miles, most people would give up before they started. If you set daily goals of one mile, they are easily attainable and you will have 1000 times more successes. You also have 1000 times more chances to improve your results.

You must have a deadline. Just saying that you want to get into shape will never work because there is no pressing time frame. If you don't have any sort of deadline, the deadline really is sometime before you die. It is human nature to drag things out and then work hard right before a deadline. With lots of short-term deadlines, you will always have that little bit of extra pressure.

Goals must be reviewed daily. You always want them to be in the forefront of your mind every day. Almost every organization has a set of goals or a mission statement, but almost nobody in any of these organizations actually knows what they are. They are usually looked at once every year or two when they are updated, but they have no impact on day-to-day activities. How many people use the excuse every year that they stopped doing their New Year's resolution because they simply forgot about it?

Setting a Resolution/Goal

First of all, nobody is perfect all the time. Accept that fact and set goals that can be achieved even if you are not always 100% on track. Secondly, all goals must be written down, reviewed and possibly refined. They should also be in a visible place so that you see them every day.

In general, all of your goals need three things: **What, When,** and **How.**

Don't set your goals too high, but don't make them too easy either. For most people, setting a one-pound weight loss goal is achievable, and over a couple of months, the results can become impressive. The more "How's" you have, the more likely you will be to accomplish your goal.

Here is an example goal.

(**What**) I will lose 30 pounds,

(**When**) in 30 weeks ending on (specific date)

(**How**) I will accomplish this by learning about weight loss and fitness through books and the F2F Radio podcast, eating 300 calories per day below my maintenance level, exercise an average of 300 calories extra per day, eating five or six small meals during the day, preparing most meals in advance, eating more "negative calorie" foods, eating a lean protein with every meal, making sure that I continue to be motivated from my support group along the way, etc.

Specific Goals

All goals should be broken down into smaller, more manageable accomplishments. It is the accomplishment of all of the smaller goals that will eventually lead you to succeed in your biggest goals.

One-Year Goals Examples could be to lose 50 pounds, lose 10% less body fat, fit into a certain size of clothing, or even be able to walk up several flights of stairs without being out of breath.

Three-Month Goals You can make huge improvements in three months. Most commercial fitness programs are designed for the three-to-four-month range. In this time frame, you can set goals like shrinking two inches off of your waist or two dress sizes smaller, or even 50% farther distance in a cycling workout. The three-month goals are more powerful than the one-year goals because of the time constraint.

Weekly and Daily Goals These are the most important and powerful goals. It is simply the accomplishment of all of these small daily goals that will allow you to achieve your ultimate goals. You don't set daily weight loss goals; you set your daily eating and exercise goals. When you follow through on your daily eating and exercise goals, the weight loss will follow. It is vitally important to plan and schedule to make certain you can accomplish these goals. For example, you can have the best intentions to eat healthy, but if you don't pack a lunch ahead of time and are forced to eat out, it probably won't happen.

Tips and Final Thoughts

Willpower will not work. Willpower is for short-term success. Long-term success requires planning, discipline and finding ways to motivate yourself every day.

Motivation will not magically happen. What motivates you will change from day to day. You have to recommit to your goals each day, tweak them to fit changes in your lifestyle and attitude, and find new ways to motivate yourself over the course of your life.

You will not always want to exercise and eat healthy. Even the most committed exerciser does not always want to do it. Know that you will have to work on it every day.

Focus on what you want on a daily basis, not what you don't want. Don't say—"I hope that I lose weight," or "I don't want to be fat," or "I hate the way that my clothes fit." Instead, flip it around to the positive and say:

- "I am getting leaner every day."
- "I am 100% responsible for my results."
- "I am a thin and fit person and I'm going to exercise today because that is what thinner and fitter people do."

THE DANGERS OF OBESITY

WHY IS IT SO BAD
TO BE FAT ANYWAY?

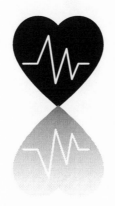

Chapter 6

"Your lifestyle—how you live, eat, emote, and think—determines your health.
To prevent disease, you may have to change how you live." —Brian Carter

DISEASES OF THE OBESE

O BESITY IS ASSOCIATED WITH CAUSING numerous diseases and conditions. Excessive body fat impairs almost every organ system in the body. Here are a few examples of the common diseases caused by obesity.

Type 2 Diabetes is a serious chronic illness that is steadily increasing in prevalence due to rising obesity rates. It leads to other complications such as blindness, kidney damage, nerve damage, limb amputations, strokes and heart disease. It is such a common and serious disease for overweight people, that it will be covered in more detail in the next chapter.

Cancer is a class of diseases characterized by cells with uncontrolled growth leading to the formation of tumors. Many types of cancer have been associated with obesity including breast, esophagus, uterus, pancreas, cervix, kidney, colon and prostate cancers. Treatments include chemotherapy, radiation therapy and surgery. Cancer is one of the leading causes of death.

Congestive Heart Failure is a condition where the heart is unable to pump enough blood to the other organs and meet the body's requirements. Blood that should be pumped out of the heart may back up into other tissues and organs, such as the lungs, causing fluid buildup. Symptoms include shortness of breath (especially when lying down), coughing, and difficulty in performing most daily activities.

Osteoarthritis is the breakdown and eventual loss of cartilage in a joint. This causes swelling, pain and limited mobility in the joint due to the bones grinding together. Obesity increases the weight bearing load and stress on the joint, which increases the rate of cartilage loss and pain.

Lymphedema is caused by a localized build up of fluid in tissues, which causes swelling in the arms or legs. The lymph fluid is unable to drain due to lack of exercise and increased body mass. This leads to heavy swollen limbs, discoloration of skin and eventual severe deformities such as elephantiasis.

Urinary Incontinence is a loss of bladder control resulting in an involuntary leakage of urine. Accumulation of excess fat in the abdominal area puts pressure on the bladder, making it more likely to leak.

Gastroesophogeal Reflux Disease (GERD) is a condition where stomach acid leaks back into the esophagus. Studies have shown that being overweight increases the chance of GERD by 50%. Symptoms include heartburn, sour taste in mouth, cough, sore throat, hoarseness and wheezing. Left untreated, this causes ulcers of the esophagus and narrowing of the esophagus.

It is always better to prevent a disease rather than try to manage a disease.

Abdominal Hernias are caused when organs bulge out between the muscles that normally hold them back inside you. This can be caused by stress on the abdominal wall due to excess fat. The organs may have the blood supply cut off and become infected.

Gallbladder Disease is a result of a sedentary lifestyle and being overweight. The liver overproduces cholesterol, which is delivered to the bile stored in the gallbladder. This produces stones that block the bile duct and produces severe pain. Treatment usually requires surgery.

Nonalcoholic Fatty Liver Disease only occurs in the obese and 75% of obese people suffer from it. It results from an accumulation of fat in liver cells. This can lead to inflammation and scarring in the liver, which can lead to liver failure.

Sleep Apnea is a chronic disorder in which you have pauses in breathing while sleeping. This results in poor sleep quality which causes excessive daytime drowsiness. One study states that 95% of sufferers are obese. Some sufferers may need to wear a mask connected to continuous positive air pressure machine when they sleep.

Gout is caused when uric acid accumulates, crystallizes and deposits in joints. Joints become painful, red and inflamed. Being overweight increases the pressure on the joints and increases the uric acid accumulation in the joints. You can treat the symptoms of gout, but it is usually a recurring problem.

Pancreatitis is inflammation of the pancreas. This organ secretes digestive enzymes and the hormone insulin. These enzymes attack the pancreas when inflammation is present causing severe pain. Long-term effects include diabetes and pancreatic cancer.

Polycystic Ovary Syndrome is a hormonal disorder among women of reproductive age. Symptoms include infertility, skin problems, and excess facial or body hair. It is also associated with insulin resistance. As little as a 10% reduction in weight can be effective in restoring regular ovulation.

Erectile Dysfunction affects a man's ability to have and sustain an erection. 80% of sufferers are overweight or obese.

The likelihood in developing all of these diseases is greatly reduced by maintaining a healthy body weight. **It is always better to prevent a disease rather than try to manage a disease.**

Chapter 7

"Strength is the capacity to break a chocolate bar into four pieces with your bare hands—and then eat just one of the pieces." —Judith Viorst

TYPE 2 DIABETES

TYPE 2 DIABETES IS ALSO known as adult-onset diabetes because it is usually developed in adulthood. Most people develop type 2 diabetes because of a lifetime of overeating and obesity. In the last decade, children are now starting to develop type 2 diabetes for the first time because of the increasing prevalence of childhood obesity. Approximately 10% of the population now has diabetes and this trend is increasing.

Type 2 diabetes is a very serious disease. Over time, it can cause vision problems, heart disease, kidney problems, nerve damage and erectile dysfunction. There are people who are permanently blind and have had limbs amputated as a result of complications of type 2 diabetes. It is possible to prevent or delay the onset of these complications once you have diabetes, but prevention of diabetes in the first place is best.

Our bodies are simply not designed to be able to handle the processing of large quantities of "bad" foods.

An abnormally high level of glucose in your blood causes the damage from type 2 diabetes. When you eat carbohydrates, they are converted into glucose. This glucose is taken out of your blood and moved into your cells to be used for energy. Someone with type 2 diabetes can't get the glucose out of their blood and moved into their cells as efficiently as they should. Insulin is the hormone that stimulates cells to absorb glucose from the blood.

Overeating and eating processed foods full of simple carbohydrates are the reasons why the diabetes epidemic is growing. Our bodies are simply not designed to be able to handle the processing of large quantities of "bad" foods.

The progression of type 2 diabetes follows two stages. **In stage one,** your cells become resistant to insulin. If you are constantly eating simple carbohydrates, your body is always flooding your bloodstream with insulin to move the glucose into your cells. Because there is always so much insulin in the blood, all of the cells become resistant to that hormone, and it no longer has the same effect as it used to.

In stage two, your body has been producing more and more insulin to try and compensate, but then it becomes unable to produce insulin.

These are generally the first symptoms that a person will develop:

- Unusual thirst
- Frequent urination
- Weight change (gain or loss)
- Extreme fatigue or lack of energy
- Blurred vision
- Frequent or recurring infections
- Cuts and bruises that are slow to heal
- Tingling or numbness in the hands or feet
- Trouble producing or maintaining an erection

It is important to recognize, however, that many people who have type 2 diabetes may display no symptoms.

The chances of developing type 2 diabetes are greatly increased if you are overweight. Other risk factors include having high cholesterol, high blood pressure or a family history of diabetes. If you are Aboriginal, Hispanic, Asian, South Asian or of African descent, you also are at a higher risk.

If you are concerned with developing type 2 diabetes, stop living the lifestyle of a person who develops type 2 diabetes. If you live the lifestyle of that thinner, healthier person, you most likely will never have to worry about it. The most important aspects of that thinner lifestyle are eating mainly healthy unprocessed foods in moderation, preferring complex carbohydrates such as oatmeal and vegetables over candy and junk food, and participating in regular physical activity.

If you are concerned with developing Type 2 diabetes, stop living the lifestyle of a person who develops type 2 diabetes.

LISTENER QUESTIONS

Q I think I might be pre-diabetic. Does that mean that I will end up with diabetes?

A You either have diabetes or you don't. There is no such medical term called "pre-diabetic" just like there is no term "pre-pregnant" or "pre-dead." If someone tells you that you are pre-diabetic, they are probably referring to metabolic syndrome and/or that you have impaired glucose tolerance.

Metabolic syndrome is diagnosed through a series of signs and symptoms. These include being overweight, having high blood pressure, high blood sugar, high cholesterol, and a sedentary lifestyle. The sad reality is that most people who have several of these characteristics will develop diabetes in the future. The more symptoms and the severity of them, will greatly increase the likelihood of a future with diabetes.

Impaired glucose tolerance is determined by your doctor through a blood test. This test is usually done one to three hours after eating and looks at the level of sugar in your blood. A person with a normal glucose tolerance test will have the same level of sugar (within a range) in their blood before and after eating. If your blood has a higher level of sugar in it after eating, your body has an impaired ability to remove that sugar.

If someone has told you that you are pre-diabetic, it is not too late to fix it.

If your impaired glucose tolerance test result is caused by overeating and obesity, there are two stages that you may pass through. In stage 1, your cells become resistant to the insulin in your body. Insulin is the hormone that takes the sugar out of your bloodstream. Because of this, your body starts producing more insulin. This leads to stage 2, where as a result of your body trying to produce more and more insulin to keep up, it begins to wear out its ability to produce insulin. When this occurs, you become diabetic.

The good news is that this is reversible. If someone has told you that you are pre-diabetic, it is not too late to fix it. By making a lifestyle change that includes eating healthier unprocessed foods, lowering your calories and increasing your exercise, you can overcome this.

FAT LOSS AND FITNESS THEORY

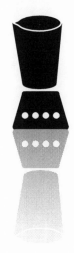

"The only thing keeping you from getting what you want is the story you keep telling yourself about why you can't have it. Break free!" —Anthony Robbins

BODY TYPES AND BODY SHAPES

ODY TYPE REFERS TO WHETHER you are a naturally skinny, muscular or heavier person (ectomorph, mesomorph, or endomorph) This has a large genetic component. Through diet and exercise, you do not have to look like your true body type though—it just takes a little more work.

A natural "skinny person" can overeat and not exercise and end up looking like an endomorph. An endomorph can look like a lean and muscular mesomorph through proper diet and exercise. Through lifestyle choices, a person can appear much different than their natural body type.

Your body shape refers to where the fat in your body naturally is distributed. This is primarily a function of the hormones in your body and your genetics. Men and women share some of the same body shapes, although some are fairly sex specific. Men tend to store fat in their lower abdomen and in their "love handles." Women tend to store fat in their hips, upper thighs and back of their arms.

These are the four basic shapes:

- **Banana or Tower Shape** Fat is distributed equally over the body. This is the typical "adolescent boy" shape. This shape is seen in both men and women.
- **Pear Shape** Fat is stored in the buttocks and legs. This is seen more in women than in men.
- **Apple Shape** This is more known as a "busty" look in women, but some men also carry their weight in their chest. The most common place that men carry their weight is in their "beer belly," which is also the most dangerous place health-wise.
- **Hourglass Shape** The "Barbie" shape. Almost only seen in women.

Can you change your body shape? The short answer is yes and no. You can drastically change the amount of fat that you have, but you can't change the places where your body naturally stores it. A person who naturally has a banana or tower shape will not develop an hourglass shape if they gain weight. Likewise a person with an hourglass shape will most likely not develop a banana or tower shape with fat loss.

"Problem areas" of fat are generally places where a person will naturally store fat first. These areas are also the last place where the fat will come off. Some "problem areas" of fat may not reduce as you would like until you are at a very low body fat percentage.

The good news: a pear shaped person can lose the fat on their thighs and buttocks. The bad news: if they gain weight, the fat goes right back to their thighs and buttocks.

LISTENER QUESTIONS

Q Do people have a natural weight that their body will naturally gravitate to?

A This is formally known as the set-point theory. It was proposed in 1982 and anecdotally has always been observed in people and animals. The basic theory is that we all have a natural weight or more specifically, fat stores, that our bodies will gravitate towards.

There is a natural variability between two very similar people, but it is a reasonable range, not hundreds of pounds of variability.

A person's body is regulated by the concept of homeostasis which keeps your body where it naturally wants to be. For example, your body likes to be at a certain temperature and you will sweat or shiver to regulate that temperature. Everyone has a slight temperature variation that is natural for their body to be at, but this variability is still within a few degrees. Nobody has a natural body temperature that is 10 or 20 degrees away from the average.

The same is believed to be true for a person's body fat percentage. There is a natural variability between two very similar people, but it is a reasonable range, not hundreds of pounds of variability. The maximum variability between people of similar sex, age and height is around 20 pounds.

So, what is that magic set-point number is for each of us? Here is a good definition:

> "Studies show that a person's weight at the set-point is optimal for efficient activity and a stable, optimistic mood. When the set point is driven too low, depression and lethargy may set in as a way of slowing the person down and reducing the number of calories expended."

Some people can have six-pack abs and seem to live a normal life. Other people will be depressed, lethargic and hungry at this low body fat percentage. Depression and lethargy are more common at the extremes.

Here is another explanation of how to find out what your natural weight should be:

> "If you eat when you are physically (not emotionally) hungry and stop (for the most part) when you are satisfied, you will find your natural weight range. This is the weight that nature intended for your body. You can maintain this weight, within a normal five to seven pound range, without dieting. There are a couple of caveats to this: If you are dieting, overeating, over-exercising or eating mainly processed foods, this will move your body away from its natural weight."

What is the scientific basis of set-point theory? There are many studies which mention set-point, but very few studies tried to look specifically at set-point. Most of the findings are from related studies that also added inferences about a person's set-point in their conclusions, but didn't specifically test for it. However most of the studies backed this theory.

So the bottom line is, yes it appears that we all have a natural set-point. If you are overeating or eating mainly processed foods, the likelihood is that you are much heavier than what your true set-point is.

Let's say that you have been eating natural foods until you are full for a few years, and have realized that your body weight has stabilized 10 pounds heavier than what you would like. Is there anything that you can do to lower your body's natural set point? The answer is yes; studies have shown that regular exercise lowers it.

Chapter 9

"The strangest secret in the world is that you become what you think about."
—Earl Nightingale.

YOUR IDEAL WEIGHT

IF YOU ARE TRYING TO lose some weight, how do you know what your goal weight should be? Depending on which method you use to determine this, your ideal weight might vary by 30 to 40 pounds or even more!

Here are the five most popular ways to determine your ideal weight:

1. The Insurance Tables of Height and Weight

In 1943, the Metropolitan Life Insurance Company introduced their standard height-weight tables for men and women. The tables were revised slightly in 1983. They were called "desirable" weights, which would indicate those persons with the lowest mortality rates. However, the phrase "ideal weight" gradually became associated with these tables in common usage, even though the word "ideal" was not specifically published with the tables.

This has turned out to be the worst way to determine your ideal weight. This is such a sweeping generalization that it may not apply to many people and may be unrealistic. The purpose of these tables was to determine life insurance risks for insurance companies; it was never designed to determine a person's ideal body weight.

2. Waist-Hip Ratio

This method might not give you an exact ideal weight, but it will give you an idea of whether you are in a healthy range or not.

To determine this, you take the circumference of your waist and then divide it by the circumference of your hips. Your answer will determine your risk of cardiovascular health problems.

MALE WAIST/HIP RATIO	FEMALE WAIST/HIP RATIO	RISK FACTOR
Less than 0.9	Less than 0.8	Low
0.9 – 0.99	0.8 – 0.89	Moderate
1.0 or over	0.9 or over	High

3. Abdominal Circumference

This is a simpler method than the Waist-Hip Ratio. All that you need is a measuring tape to measure the largest part of your abdomen. This method works regardless of your body type.

This measurement is directly related to the most dangerous fat—abdominal, intra-organ fat. This leads to metabolic syndrome, diabetes, hypertension, premature cardiovascular disease etc.

For a male, the ideal abdominal circumference is less than 37 inches. Subtract two inches for females. These numbers are one to two inches less for Southeast Asians.

4. Body Mass Index (BMI)

The BMI relates your height to your weight. Technically, these are the formulas used:

English BMI Formula
BMI = (weight in pounds / (height in inches) x (height in inches)) x 703
Metric BMI Formula
BMI = (weight in kilograms / (height in meters) x (height in meters))

If you do a simple search on the Internet for "BMI calculator," you will be able to find many resources where you can plug in your figures and it will do the calculation for you.

Health authorities worldwide mostly agree that:

- People with a BMI of less than 18.5 are underweight.
- A BMI of between 18.5 and 25 is ideal.
- Somebody with a BMI between 25 and 30 is classed as overweight.
- A person with a BMI over 30 is obese.

The BMI is one of the most commonly used tools, and it can give you ballpark information, but it is prone to many errors. When comparing large populations of people, such as North Americans to Europeans, it can clearly show obesity trends, but it is not ideal for comparing individuals.

One obvious problem is that there is no distinction between men and women. Men and women of the same height should not weigh the same amount! A man has more muscle than a woman and therefore will weigh more than a woman of the same height. On the BMI scale, this man will be considered less healthy than the woman because his BMI will be higher.

The BMI is one of the most commonly used tools, and it can give you ballpark information, but it is prone to many errors.

People of the same sex may also get inaccurate results based on their personal body compositions. A very weak person with very little muscle mass and a large proportion of fat can easily fit within the "healthy" BMI range. A naturally strong person with more muscle mass and a low level of body fat can be considered overweight using the BMI scale.

5. The Muscle-Fat Ratio (Body Fat Percentage)

We consider people to be obese when they have a higher level of body fat. You are not obese because you have more muscle, bone density, tendons, ligaments, water weight etc. The best way to determine your ideal weight is actually not looking at your weight, but by looking at your body fat percentage.

According to the former U.S Surgeon General Dr. Koop, "One's body fat percentage is superior to the currently accepted body mass index (BMI), as a measure of healthy weight." His advisory to physicians states that "body fat percentage is as significant an indicator of health status as blood pressure and blood cholesterol levels. In fact, body fat percentage is a more direct assessment of healthy weight because it is able to distinguish fat from muscle."

The American Council on Exercise recommends the following percentages:

CATEGORY	MEN	WOMEN
Athletes	6-13%	14-20%
Healthy and Fit	14-17%	21-24%
Acceptable	18-25%	25-31%
Overweight	26-37%	32-41%
Obese	Greater than 38%	Greater than 42%

What would we suggest that you do to find out your ideal weight?

1. Use BMI to get an initial ballpark figure. Use the BMI of 25, which is the upper range of "ideal." So now you have your starting point to set your initial tentative goal.

2. Once you start to approach this weight, then switch to body fat percentage. Use one of the many ways that you can measure your body fat. We suggest a body fat scale that does both your weight and your body fat at the same time.

LISTENER QUESTIONS

Q Are you destined to be fat if you have bad genes?

A There is no question that people are different genetically. Properties such as hair color, height, shoe size and hairiness are clearly obvious. People also have different body types. Some people are naturally more muscular, some are thinner and others naturally have higher body fat levels.

Certain characteristics you are born with such as eye color. There is nothing that you can do about your eye color. You can wear colored contacts to cover over your true eye color, but you can't change your genes. Many of our genes need to interact with our environment to be expressed. This is the "nature versus nurture" reality.

For example, let's take heart disease. Your doctor will often ask you about your family's history of heart disease. Your doctor will ask you this to find out if you have "bad genes." If it turns out that all of your relatives have suffered from heart disease, that does not mean that you will die from heart disease. That only means that you have a higher potential to suffer from heart disease. Your lifestyle will have a greater impact on the chances of you dying from it.

With poor genes, if you live an unhealthy lifestyle and eat poorly, the chances are much higher than the general population that you will develop heart disease.

> You may have a predisposition to have more body fat, but it is the combination of your environment and your lifestyle that will make you fat.

If you live a healthy lifestyle, your chances might not be any greater than the general population. The point is, just because your grandparents died from heart attacks when they were in their 40s, this isn't a guarantee that you will as well. Eat healthy, make sure that you keep your weight and your blood pressure under control, and the chances are extremely high that you will live into your 70s or 80s.

The same thing is true with your chances of becoming obese. You may have a predisposition to have more body fat, but it is the combination of your environment and your lifestyle that will make you fat. Some people will have an easier time gaining fat than others, but that does not mean that you are destined to be fat. Your lifestyle choices—what you choose to eat and the level of physical activity that you choose to do, will have a much greater impact on obesity than your genes.

There is not a single person in the world that weighs 400 pounds and does not eat more food than a 150-pound person. That 400-pound person may have an easier time gaining fat, but they are still choosing to eat many more calories on average every single day to get there.

Chapter 10

"Success seems to be largely a matter of hanging on after others have let go."
—*William Feather*

WHY CAN'T I LOSE WEIGHT?

F A PERSON IS STRANDED on a desert island for years at a time with very little food to eat, they will lose weight. Even if that person has struggled for years trying to lose weight, when they are rescued years later, they will have considerably less fat on them. We all know this is true.

100% of people who follow a sensible exercise and eating program will lose weight. They may not lose weight at the same rate, but every person can reach their healthy weight.

Many people find that they are struggling to lose weight, but 95% of those people are struggling because of simple errors that can be fixed! Here are the top eight errors that people make in fat loss.

1. Education

Most people learn all about nutrition in elementary school, but they soon forget all of that knowledge after being bombarded with other advice from the mass media. By the time they reach adulthood, the majority of all information that people remember about nutrition and exercise, they learn from pop culture. They learn how to train from "Rocky" movies, and learn how to diet from talk shows like "Oprah" or "The View" or even worse, weight loss competition shows like "The Biggest Loser." Often this information is blatantly wrong and often distorted for the purpose of entertainment.

> Survey after survey shows that over 90% of people underestimate the calories in food.

2. Food Reasons

This is the biggest reason why people don't seem to be able to lose fat. Survey after survey shows that over 90% of people underestimate the calories in food. In one survey, the average estimate of a Subway meal was between 350-400 calories when it was actually over 1000. If those people continued to overestimate their daily calories by 600 each day, that would keep them from losing over five pounds per month!

Some people refuse to count calories and prefer to use "point systems" or rules of thumb to track how much they are eating during the day. It doesn't matter how you keep track, you just have to have a caloric deficit to lose fat.

A food journal is a very good tool to keep you on track. If you don't track calories, you can still track portions. Make sure that you watch out for hidden calories such as sugar in beverages, condiments such as ketchup, or even supplements. Sampling food while cooking catches a lot of people, as does eating at night, snacking and of course the candy dish at work.

3. Exercise Reasons

We assume that you exercise. The biggest exercise failure doesn't have to do with exercising itself, it's wasting all of the fat loss benefits by eating after. Many over-estimate the amount of calories they are burning during exercise and then over-compensate as a reward after. Sports drinks are also a big problem because they can contain a lot of calories. The calories listed on the sides are usually per serving, but the bottle may contain two or three servings, so be careful.

Previous crash diets can have a lasting effect on your metabolism.

To get the full benefit out of exercise, it should be challenging—you should break a sweat! However, make sure that you slowly build up the intensity of your workouts over time so that you reduce the risk of injury or over training. If you are looking to burn extra calories to help reduce fat, do the exercises that use the most combination of muscles and the largest muscles in the body. Cycling is good because it uses your legs, walking on a treadmill on a steep incline is better because it uses more leg muscles, and using an elliptical trainer is even better because it uses both your legs and your arms.

4. Damage From Previous Diets

Previous crash diets can have a lasting effect on your metabolism. Each time that a person goes on a low calorie diet, they end up losing muscle mass. For every pound of muscle mass that they lose, they damage their metabolism by 30 to 50 calories.

If a person loses 10 pounds very quickly and then gains it back, they now have to eat less to maintain their original weight than in the first place before their diet. Because of this, every time they go on a diet, it gets harder and harder to keep the weight off.

This damage can be fixed through a good eating program and dedication to a resistance training program to regain lost muscle.

5. Hitting a Plateau

When you hit a weight loss plateau, it is either caused from eating too few calories, or by simply dieting over a long time without a break. A plateau is simply when your body notices that you are losing weight and thinks that it is starting to starve.

You cannot break through a plateau by eating less or exercising more—you must do the opposite.

Dieting is hard on your body. The simple solution is to eat more calories. Eat at your maintenance calories or even a few hundred more per day for a few weeks to convince your body that you are not starving. You might gain a pound or two, but once you give your body a break and remove the stress of dieting for a little while, when you lower your calories again, it will start releasing fat again.

6. Emotional Reasons

Almost all people are emotional eaters to some extent. We are all taught at a young age that food and happiness can be combined together. Good tasting food simply makes us feel good. This has been true since your first birthday party with cake and every family get-together since then almost always has a meal.

The first step is to identify if you are eating for other reasons than hunger.

The problem arises when people eat when they are not truly hungry. If you eat to feel better emotionally, as a coping habit, out of boredom, to reduce stress or to "fill the hollow feeling in your stomach" when you are upset, this is a recipe for weight gain.

The first step is to identify if you are eating for other reasons than hunger. The second step is to substitute other things in your life to alleviate those emotional concerns.

7. Motivational Reasons

Nobody can motivate you to do anything in the long run. You must truly want to be healthy in order to change your lifestyle to that thinner and healthier person. Here are some quick tips to improve your own motivation.

- Come up with powerful reasons as to why you want to lose fat. What would happen if you didn't lose the weight?
- The pain of **not** losing weight should be **more** painful than losing weight.
- Goal setting is truly the key. With daily, weekly, and monthly goals you will have many successes to continually keep you on track and provide you with daily motivation.

8. Medical Reasons

There are a variety of medical reasons why it may be difficult to lose weight. Polycystic ovary syndrome (PCOS) effects 5% of women, many people have hormone problems such as hypothyroidism, and even some medications have been associated with weight gain. A regular checkup or physical with your doctor is the best course of action to deal with these issues.

LISTENER QUESTIONS

Q How do I figure out the exact number of calories I burn each day?

A There are several calculators that try to calculate how many calories you burn in a day based on similar assumptions. The biggest factor that determines the speed of someone's metabolism is the amount of muscle mass that they have. Unfortunately, these calculators usually only ask for a person's age, sex, height and weight. Based on those factors, the calculators make estimations on the amount of muscle that the average person in your situation has.

The biggest factor that determines the speed of someone's metabolism is the amount of muscle mass that they have.

All calculators first figure out your Basal Metabolic Rate, which is the amount of calories that your body would burn if you were in a coma without any voluntary movement.

The second step is to estimate the average amount of activity that you do on a daily basis. This activity estimation is then multiplied with your BMR, to estimate your total caloric burn.

So for example, if a person's BMR is exactly 1000 calories per day and they are a total "couch potato," you can estimate their total calories. The sedentary activity multiplier is 1.2. Multiplying 1000 by 1.2 would estimate that person could eat 1200 calories per day to maintain their weight. But if that person worked out very hard and also had a very hard physical job, their activity multiplier might be as high as 1.9. So that means that they could eat 1900 calories per day to maintain their weight.

Everyone falls somewhere in the middle, and these are all approximations. The "light workout" level, which is one to three times per week, is 1.375 times your BMR. In reality, we know that if two people work out three times per week, there is no real chance that they will each burn the same number of calories during those two workouts. Think of two people in a group fitness class; not everyone does the same intensity or effort during the class, so not everyone will have the same caloric benefit.

These numbers are always going to be estimations. Use them to set approximate, but realistic levels of how many calories you should be eating. Monitor how you are doing and then adjust them slightly as needed based on your results.

You can get pretty close to figuring out exactly how many calories you burn, but it takes careful tracking to figure it out. We suggest that you use the formulas to get close. Then track how many calories you are eating and carefully monitor your weight. When your weight stabilizes, you will know the true amount of calories that you burn each day.

> Ultimately, it is calories in versus calories out.

Ultimately, it is calories in versus calories out. Know your approximate numbers. If you are not losing any weight at all, decrease the calories you eat and increase the calories you burn a little bit more. When you hit your goal weight, increase your calories a little bit at a time until your weight stabilizes.

Chapter 11

"Why doesn't someone do something about how fat I am?"
—*Dori from Traineo*

THE BASICS OF BODY FAT

I F YOU HEAD TO THE magazine rack at the grocery store and look at the fitness magazines, you would think they had the end all, be all answer to shrinking your belly. It seems the magazine publishing industry knows exactly what you want. Unfortunately they can't deliver you a flat belly in four weeks.

Here is a quick primer on body fat. There are two types of fat that you should be concerned about:

Visceral fat is the fat that exists around your organs to cushion them. This is the worst kind of body fat and is associated with metabolic syndrome and a higher risk of type 2 diabetes and heart disease.

Subcutaneous fat is the fat beneath the skin. If visceral fat is the cushion for your organs, subcutaneous fat is your body's shock absorber. This is the fat that helps cushion you against trauma. It is also the fat that is burned during periods of high activity. In other words, if you want to burn off your subcutaneous fat, you need to exercise.

Men and women tend to accumulate fat in different places. Men typically carry more fat in their abdomen, which is generally the dangerous visceral type. Women typically accumulate fat on the thighs and buttocks.

Depending on your genetics, fat deposits can show up almost anywhere on a person's body. Other popular spots are the inside portion of the knee, the upper arm, the lower back and the chest. Also, particular ethnic groups will accumulate fat in different places. For example, Asian adults are more prone to visceral and central obesity than those of European decent and Mediterranean women are more likely to gain fat on their outer thighs.

Fat is shed differently from person to person, but it tends to go first from the most recent place it appeared. If your belly started gaining first—this will be the very last place for the fat to disappear from. A person might be losing fat and not see a difference in their circumference measurements if that fat is coming off of their fingers and calves first.

Despite what you may have heard in advertisements and diet books, there is no way to target a certain area to lose fat. You cannot just target belly fat. Your belly will decrease as your overall body fat decreases.

There is no way to target a certain area to lose fat.

The visceral fat is the fat between the organs, tends to react more quickly to diet and will initially shrink faster than subcutaneous fat. That is good news for reducing your health risks, but keep in mind that subcutaneous fat makes up 80% of your body fat. The subcutaneous fat responds best to exercise.

Is a flatter stomach possible? Yes, but only as part of an overall reduction in body fat.

Can you get a flat stomach in four weeks? No, probably not, but that visceral fat in your abdomen will be among the first to go as you start eating like that thinner person you want to become.

Can you get there by just dieting? Dieting alone will get you part way to your goal, but will not completely get you there. You need to exercise and create a caloric deficit by way of exercise to shrink those fat cells over your entire body. By doing this, over time, you will achieve a flatter stomach as well as lower your overall body fat. The reality is it is not going to happen overnight and it will be hard work.

LISTENER QUESTIONS

Q Can you grow back fat cells after liposuction?

A Liposuction is not an effective means of weight loss. The most amount of fat that can be safely removed in one surgery is only six to eight pounds. According to plastic surgeons, liposuction is for the purpose of changing the shape of a person's body, not for significant amounts of fat loss. According to Liposuction.com, these are the facts about liposuction and the realistic expectations that you can expect:

1. If you do not gain any weight after liposuction, the fat that was removed will not grow back.

2. If you do gain weight after liposuction, that fat generally first goes to the areas with the highest concentration of fat cells. If a woman has removed fat cells from her thighs and legs, any new fat that is gained will proportionally go to other places with a higher concentration such as her breasts, back and arms.

3. The areas that have been treated with liposuction will still accumulate fat, but generally to a lesser degree. The fat will be distributed differently around the body.

4. The fat cells that were removed by liposuction can come back if a person gains a significant amount of weight. With a small weight gain, existing fat cells simply get bigger by accumulating more fat within the existing cell. However, with an increase of more than 10% of body weight, one can expect new fat cell development in all areas of the body, including areas previously treated by liposuction.

LISTENER QUESTIONS

Q Why do most people who lose weight gain it all back?

A When a person loses weight incredibly fast, many people find that impressive. Granted, they have worked extremely hard and made many sacrifices to achieve their weight loss goals and their efforts are impressive.

Statistically, almost every single dieter who loses weight extremely fast will not have any long-term success in keeping it off. A person who loses 100 pounds in five months will probably have greater than 99% chance of gaining the majority, if not all of their weight back within two years.

Here are the reasons why people seem to always gain their weight back after dieting:

1. **When people lose weight too quickly, they lose muscle mass.**
    Muscle is the key to your metabolism. If you lose muscle while dieting,

your metabolism slows down. With a slower metabolism, it is even harder to keep the weight off. If a person returned to their old eating habits, they would not only gain all of their weight back, but they would gain even more.

2. **Diets don't work because they are only temporary.** People think of diets as weeks or months of deprivation and hunger and look forward to when the diet is over. Once they are off their diet, they return back to the lifestyle of a heavier person and once again become that heavier person.

3. **Diets are simply too hard.** When you diet strictly for a long time, it takes a lot of willpower and determination. The vast majority of dieters reach their goal weight for only a matter of days or weeks. After they have accomplished their goal, they lose all of their motivation. When people try so hard to reach one specific number on a scale, they don't know what to do when they reach it. The new goal of maintaining their weight loss usually doesn't cross their mind as they go out to eat sinful and decadent foods to celebrate their weight loss!

> Why do people regain? Once they are off their diet, they return back to the lifestyle of a heavier person and once again become that heavier person.

4. **Denial of foods causes people to crave them more.** All foods can fit into a fat loss program if they are eaten in moderation. For example, people who are "chocoholics" tend to binge and give up on diets after a few weeks of abstinence.

5. **Undereating will always lead to overeating.** Willpower only works in the short term. Over an extended time of severe caloric restriction, the psychological factors will add up and the desire to gorge and eat more food will win out.

6. **Lifestyle modification is the solution.** The real key is to change your lifestyle to that of a thinner person *for good*. If your attitude is to lose 15 pounds this month for an upcoming wedding, most likely in six months, all of your weight will be back. If your attitude is to never diet again because you adopt that "thinner person's lifestyle," you will not need to diet for any more weddings in the future.

Chapter 12

"You cannot improve what you cannot measure—just make sure you are measuring the right thing." —Jeff Ainslie

MUSCLE VERSUS FAT

W HEN YOU ARE TRYING TO lose "weight," the ultimate goal is to lose fat, not muscle mass. The faster you lose weight, the more of that weight loss comes from muscle instead of fat.

Muscle is the key to your metabolism, and if you lose muscle, you will slow down your metabolism. With a sluggish body, you naturally burn less calories per day, which means you have to eat less every day to maintain your weight. This also means that it will be much easier to gain weight again in the future.

Your muscles are the most metabolically active cells in your body; they burn a lot of calories every day even if you don't do anything. Fat sits passively on your body compared to muscle. If you were in a coma and didn't move, a single pound of muscle would burn around 14 calories per day, a pound of fat burns about five calories per day.

Each pound of muscle really burns between 30 and 50 calories per day.

You are living and moving around and using those muscles, so each pound of muscle really burns between 30 and 50 calories per day. A pound of fat will always burn around five calories per day.

Why is this such an important fact?

For every pound of muscle that you lose through dieting, you will damage your metabolism by 30 to 50 calories per day. If you lose 10 pounds of "weight," but five pounds of that weight loss was muscle, you have damaged your metabolism by at least 150 calories per day. That means that you will have to eat 150 calories less per day now to maintain your weight. What happens if you don't eat 150 calories less per day? Well, after a few years that will add up to around 25 pounds of extra fat.

This is one of the main reasons why people end up yo-yo dieting. Every time that they go on an unhealthy diet, they tend to lose muscle mass, which slows down their metabolism, which makes it harder to keep the weight off each time they lose weight.

If your body thinks that it is starving (for example eating under 1500 calories per day), it will do whatever it can to slow down its metabolism. Your body doesn't know that you are on a diet; it is just trying to survive. The best way that it knows to slow down its own metabolism is to get rid of metabolically active muscle because it uses so much energy. In starvation mode, your body doesn't burn just fat, it is also digesting your muscle.

Everyone's goal should be to eat the most amount of food and be lean and healthy. By dieting too fast and undereating, you now have to eat less food per day than what you should be able to. Your metabolism will stay this slow until you do some serious training to gain that lost muscle back.

It is very easy to lose fat without losing muscle at the same time. The key is simply going slow. The fastest that you would ever want to lose weight would be one to two pounds or 1% of your body weight each week.

LISTENER QUESTIONS

Q Why does your body eat its own muscle instead of fat if you eat too little?

A Your body is very adept at staying alive. If you are very cold you will start to shiver, if you are hot you will start to sweat, if you are frightened, your body will release adrenalin.

If your body is in a life-threatening condition, it has many strategies to help it recover and stay alive. With a traumatic event, people go into shock and they disassociate from the experience and may not even feel the pain of a serious injury. When your body is recovering from surgery, most people sleep most of the day because their body knows that this is the best way for it to recover.

When you eat too little food, that is a potential life threatening condition for your body. It knows that eventually, it may die if you continue to eat at those low calorie levels. It quickly goes into what is known as starvation mode where it does whatever it can to stay alive on this low level of calories.

The best way that it knows to slow down your metabolism is by getting rid of some of your muscle mass. Each pound of muscle burns between 30 and 50 calories per day, while a pound of fat burns five calories per day. If it is worried about staying alive, it is going to get rid of the most metabolically active tissues first that require the most energy. It is true that fat has a lot more energy in it than muscle mass, but your body is in a panic right now.

When you eat too little food, that is a potential life-threatening condition for your body.

To get it out of a panic, you need to eat more food. When you do that, your body will realize that it isn't starving and with a moderate reduction in calories, it will start losing fat again.

If you eat below your basal metabolic rate, you guarantee that some of your weight loss will come from muscle mass instead of fat. For most people, their BMR is at least 1500 calories.

Chapter 13

"A week of neglect could cost you a year of repair."
—Jim Rohn

BREAKING WEIGHT LOSS PLATEAUS

ONE OF THE MOST COMMON questions/problems/concerns from our listeners is what to do when their weight loss seems to stall. It can be an extremely frustrating time for dieters. Many have gone months eating at their goal calorie levels and regularly exercising and have consistently lost weight week after week. Then the weight loss stops for weeks or months with no obvious reason.

This is one situation where if you follow your instincts, you will do exactly the wrong thing and make your weight loss plateau worse.

Most people think that they just are not trying hard enough. They will eat even less and increase their exercise to try to kick start their weight loss. By doing this, they only end up making things harder on themselves and suffer needlessly. You cannot use willpower or determination to get out of a plateau, you don't need to work harder, only smarter.

To break out of a plateau, you must eat more. To truly break free, you need to eat at your maintenance level or even a couple hundred calories more per day for a few weeks.

A weight loss plateau is caused by one of two reasons. The most common cause is known as underfeeding. This happens when you are not eating enough calories on a daily basis. The second common cause is from long-term dieting. In both cases, the body has gone into a starvation response and is simply slowing down its metabolism to keep from losing all of its fat and dying! Your body has no idea that this reduction in food isn't going to be permanent.

> If you eat too few calories, your body panics to keep itself at the status quo.

Dieting is stressful on your body. If you eat too few calories, your body panics to keep itself at the status quo. If you eat below your Basal Metabolic Rate, that is a guarantee that your body will quickly go into "starvation mode." An average man's

BMR is around 1900 calories, an average woman's is around 1500. Even if you are only eating at a moderate reduction in calories, after several months, your body will realize that it has been losing fat and can move into a starvation response.

The simple way to get out of a plateau is to remove the stress from dieting long enough to convince your body that it is not at risk of starvation. Then when you reduce your calories again, you will begin to lose fat once more.

Many people are concerned that if they eat at their maintenance calories for a few weeks, they may end up gaining weight. This may happen, but it may be necessary to fix your stalled metabolism. In a month or two, you will be much farther ahead.

Here are some tips that will help you avoid plateaus:

- Only do a moderate restriction in calories of no more than 500 per day.
- Make sure that a portion of your fat loss is a result from doing exercise and activities, not only caloric restriction.
- Take some time off from dieting every once in a while. A cheat meal once a week or even a cheat weekend once a month will help you in the long run.
- Don't do the exact same workouts day after day. Make sure that you are continually changing you activities so that your body does not become adapted to any routine.
- Make sure that you are eating often throughout the day. Try to eat a meal or healthy snack every three to four hours and never skip meals.

LISTENER QUESTIONS

Q Could my weight loss plateau become permanent? If I didn't make any changes to my calorie intake or my workout routine, wouldn't my plateau work itself out over time and eventually my weight loss start up again?

A A plateau is really just your body responding to its survival instinct in a physical way. If it thinks that you are in a famine and starving, it will do whatever it takes to slow down your metabolism.

Once you take away your body's perceived stress about starvation, it will loosen up and you will start losing fat again. We have been giving this advice for the past three years, and regularly receive emails from many people who report that increasing their calories has broken them out of plateaus that were months or years long. A common sentiment from these people is "Why did I make myself suffer for so long?"

Could your plateau become permanent? The short answer is yes, or at least you can permanently slow your metabolism down. When your body thinks that it is slowly starving and is trying to slow its own metabolism, the best way that it knows to do this is by reducing your muscle mass. For every pound of muscle that your body digests, you metabolism will be slower until you spend months or years in a gym to gain that muscle back. In fact, the only reason that men burn more calories per day and have an easier time losing weight than women, is because they have more muscle mass.

> For every pound of muscle that your body digests, you metabolism will be slower until you spend months or years in a gym to gain that muscle back.

To answer the question about whether with a lot of patience, your body will break out of a plateau if you keep struggling and eating those low calories, the answer is no.

There is almost no chance of that happening. The reason is that your body has found its homeostasis level where it can maintain its weight on low calories. **Your body isn't all of a sudden going to forget its own survival instinct and start losing fat if it thinks it is in a famine.**

If you have been eating 1500 calories per day and haven't lost any weight in six months, why would you expect things to change in the future? If your maintenance level is 2400 calories, eat at least 2400 calories a day for a couple of weeks. Then lower your calories again later.

Losing body fat isn't all about willpower—sometimes you just need to work smarter and work with your body, not against it.

Chapter 14

"If you don't have time to do it right you must have time to do it over." —Unknown

EVERYTHING YOU NEED TO KNOW ABOUT WEIGHT LOSS SUPPLEMENTS

WEIGHT LOSS SUPPLEMENTS ARE EXTREMELY popular and consumers spend billions of dollars per year on them. If you search for "diet drugs" on the Internet, you will find thousands of sites that praise the benefits of these products. Most of these sites are simply disguised sales sites for these supplements, and are loaded with fake consumer reviews. So how is the average person able to tell the difference between products, separate the hype, and find out if any supplements even help you lose fat?

In the United States, the Food and Drug Administration regulates supplements to the same degree that they would regulate a loaf of bread.

First, it is important to understand that prescription diet drugs and weight loss supplements are not the same thing. Diet drugs are regulated, they "claim to cure, mitigate, or treat a disease," and have scientific evidence that they work. They follow regulations to ensure quality control and that the ingredients stated are actually in the drugs and in the advertised ratios. Weight loss supplements are classified in the same category as food products. They are considered to be dietary supplements and are intended to supply nutrients that are missing or not consumed in sufficient quantity in a person's diet.

In the United States, the Food and Drug Administration regulates supplements to the same degree that they would regulate a loaf of bread. Supplement manufacturers do not have to ensure quality control, and are not required to prove the safety or effectiveness of their products. The FDA can take action only after a dietary supplement has been proven harmful. Ephedra is an example of a supplement that caused serious cardiovascular effects and several deaths. Because of this, it was pulled from the market.

Even though supplements are not considered to be drugs, they can interact with other supplements and medications. In fact, some supplements can counteract the effects of some prescription medications. For example, Ginkgo Biloba can interact with blood thinning medications.

Most people purchase supplements from a supplement store and receive supplement advice from the clerks who work there. Most of these clerks make a commission on every bottle of supplements that they sell, and are educated about those supplements from promotional material provided by the manufacturers. Promotional material is designed to sell products, not necessarily provide factual and non-biased information. Even though a supplement store may seem to be the logical place to buy supplements, it may be the worst place to find out factual information about supplements.

> Scientifically, if you want to double or triple the results of weight loss supplements all that you have to do is choose to eat one less piece of bread per day.

The best place to get informed advice about any supplements is from a pharmacist. A pharmacist has years of specific training on drugs and their interactions. As well, promotional materials do not bias them. They are trained to look for possible interactions and base their recommendations on scientific principles and scientific evidence.

There are many popular weight loss supplements on the market today. Here are some interesting facts about them:

- The most popular weight loss supplements are different in different geographic locations and from store to store.
- The most popular ones are the ones that are the most advertised and marketed in a particular area.
- The popularity of a weight loss supplement has nothing to do with how well it helps you lose weight, or even if it helps you at all. They are based on hype.

Supplements do have ingredients that can have a physiological impact on your body. The most common chemicals in weight loss supplements are bitter orange, caffeine, and chromium. These chemicals may not be specifically listed in the ingredients, but will be a component in many of the herbs listed. The goal is to temporarily speed up a person's metabolism so they will either burn more calories or reduce hunger. Many of the most popular weight loss supplements have the same caffeine impact of dozens of cups of coffee or cans of soda. Common side effects are jitters, shakes, headaches, anxiety, heart problems, and insomnia.

The most important question is whether any weight loss supplements will have an impact on your weight loss. Unfortunately, the independent scientific studies do not show any great impact on weight loss in the participants. Some of the latest studies have been looking at the effects of chromium on weight loss. The most promising studies show up to a two-pound weight loss in two to three months. That is nowhere near the claimed results advertised!

The conclusion about weight loss supplements is that they do not live up to their promises. They are an extra cost financially, and will clearly not have any significant impact on weight loss. Scientifically, if you want to double or triple the results of weight loss supplements without the headaches, jitters, shakes etc, all that you have to do is choose to eat one less piece of bread per day.

LISTENER QUESTIONS

Q Do you really need supplements or meal replacements for weight loss?

A This is a very common question from people who are on commercial diet programs. Most of these programs recommend or require their clients to purchase their brands of supplements. In some cases, the recommended supplements will cost hundreds of dollars per month.

In almost every instance, it is better to eat "real food" instead of a meal replacement shake or bar.

In every single case, you do not have to take the required supplements or meal replacements for weight loss. All that you need to ensure is that you are eating fewer calories than what you burn to lose fat.

In the last few years, the diet industry discovered a new way to make even more money than just selling diet programs. They started making and selling their own diet supplements—everything from meal replacements, vitamins, nutrition bars, fiber supplements etc. Many commercial diet programs make the majority of their profits by selling supplements.

Take a look at the Atkins Diet. You can buy Atkins vitamins and Atkins meal replacement bars. The same is even true for diets such as the Zone and South

Beach diets. Even the regular "Diet Centres" such as Nutrisystem and Jenny Craig sell their own supplements and vitamins.

This is such a lucrative business that companies are now creating supplements and meal replacements and **then** creating the diet program in order to sell them.

The most well-known diet that did this was *Body For Life* by Bill Phillips. Bill Phillips is the owner of the giant supplement company EAS which makes the meal replacement called Myoplex. It is no surprise that the suggested menus in this program list two meals per day of Myoplex!

In almost every instance, it is better to eat "real food" instead of a meal replacement shake or bar. To digest real food, your body burns calories in the digestion process, so your net calories are lower than the actual calories that you just ate. This is great if you are concerned with losing weight, not to mention that real food isn't as painful on your pocketbook!

Many of these diet programs that are based on supplement products are not necessarily bad. If the program suggests a balanced diet, there is nothing wrong with eating an occasional supplement product. There is also nothing wrong with eating a sensible balanced meal instead of a suggested supplement and still have success on any program.

Unless you are planning to continue to take all of these extra supplements and meal replacement products for the rest of your life after you reach your goal, it would be wise not to become dependent on them for long-term weight loss.

Chapter 15

"Short term thinking is the social disease of our time."
—Norman Lear

FASTING AND DETOX PLANS

MOST DETOX PLANS ARE REALLY nothing more than fasting for a week or 10 days with minimal intake of calories. One of the perceived benefits of going through a detox program is that people will see some weight loss benefits.

The problem is, compared to **any** weight loss program, detox and fasting has the lowest success rate and the fastest rebound weight gain.

Compared to **any** weight loss program, detox and fasting has the lowest success rate and the fastest rebound weight gain.

When a person goes on a detox or a fast, there are immediate psychological and physiological consequences. Starving yourself causes intense cravings for food and most people will over-compensate long after the fast is done. It also slows down your metabolism, which can cause permanent damage that can take months or years to repair.

Here are some reasons why fasting and detox programs should never be done for the purpose of weight loss:

1. **Fasting to detox your body simply does not make logical sense.** Your body eliminates toxins through your liver 24 hours a day. When you fast, it quickly slows down your metabolism. This causes all of your metabolic processes to slow down, including your liver. Therefore it would take longer for your body to process and remove any toxins. Just stop eating processed food! Start eating clean, healthy, unprocessed foods instead of putting yourself through all of that hunger and deprivation.

2. **Starving yourself does not make you healthier or make you feel healthy.** Think of it this way, if you are being chased by a grizzly bear while out camping, is your body going to be functioning properly while near the end of a fast? No—you will be mentally and physically sluggish. You will not be healthier after a fast, you will be in recovery.

3. **Sumo wrestlers use periodic fasting to gain weight.** They do not eat all day long, they eat one big meal in the morning and one at night with usually 12 hours of fasting in between. Over the centuries, they have realized that not eating for stretches often helps them gain fat.

4. **When you do start eating again, you body will be a fat storing machine for the next while!** Thousands of years ago when food was in short supply, it was beneficial that our metabolisms could slow down quickly, so we could survive without food for a while. When food became plentiful again, fat was stored at a very accelerated rate to prepare for the next famine.

   As well, if you lose even a tiny bit of muscle while you fast, your metabolism will not return to where it was until you put in the gym time to gain that muscle back. You can't fight your body's mental desire to eat. Undereating will always lead to overeating.

   > Anything that you do that is temporary in dieting gives you temporary results.

5. **Our philosophy is that if you want permanent weight loss, you simply have to live the life of that thinner person that you want to become.** Thinner, healthy people **do not f**ast for the purpose of maintaining their weight. They simply eat and exercise at the average level that keeps them at their current weight. Anything that you do that is temporary in dieting gives you temporary results.

6. **There is no such thing as a "jump start" on weight loss.** Many programs start off with an intense week, so that people will think that they have lost a significant amount of weight quickly at the start and may be more motivated to continue. It isn't real weight loss, and most people find that they quickly plateau.

   What really happens in the first few days is a loss of water weight. This is caused by two things. First, you will be eating less processed foods and therefore, less salt. Salt causes your body to retain a higher level of water in your tissues. When you lower your salt intake, you water level will quickly decrease. Second, when the glycogen in your muscles is used up, water comes out of the muscle as well. When you start to eat again, your muscles are begging for glycogen fuel again, and the water comes right back into your muscles along with it.

7. **The idea that fasting is normal or healthy for people in our modern society is potentially dangerous.** This argument is seen on pro-anorexia and pro-bulimia forums. Periodic fasting, for almost all anorexics, is the "gateway drug" that starts them thinking that this is normal. Not eating is not normal or healthy. Fasting to lose weight is a sign of desperation without knowledge or understanding of the consequences.

LISTENER QUESTIONS

Q Why do people get fatter as they get older?

A Let's face it, as you age your body not only ages—it also changes. How much you actually weigh becomes less and less of an issue for your overall appearance.

> The fact that people naturally lose muscle as they age is also the reason that people put on weight as they age.

Does a 95-year-old woman physically look the same as when she was 16 if she weighs the same amount? Of course not, and we are not just talking about wrinkles. If you compared her arms and her legs, there would be a huge difference in tone and shape. The older person would also be larger and softer—they would not be able to fit into the same clothes even though they weighed the same amount.

Here is the reason: **After age 30, you naturally lose six pounds of muscle every decade.** If you weigh the same at age 30 and 40, you will have a higher body fat percentage at age 40. You would have six pounds less muscle and six pounds more fat. A pound of fat is many times larger in volume than a pound of muscle. A pound of muscle also naturally burns 30 to 50 calories per day, whereas a pound of fat only burns five calories.

The fact that people naturally lose muscle as they age is also the reason that people put on weight as they age. Here is an example that will demonstrate how the average man can gain 60 to 100 pounds in his lifetime without ever overeating.

Here is an average man (numbers are rounded for clarity):

- 30 years old, 5'10", 180 pounds and moderate activity. He will burn about 2500 calories per day to maintain his weight.
- At age 40, if he has now lost five pounds of muscle, he will need to eat 2300 calories per day to maintain his weight (five pounds of muscle x 40 calories per day average = 200). He can easily gain 10 pounds per year, if he continues to eat the same amount of calories that he could eat at age 30.
- At age 50, he has now lost another five pounds of muscle. He will now have to eat 2100 calories per day to maintain his weight. He can continue to easily gain another 10 pounds per year, if he continues to eat like he did when he was 30.

So what is the point? If at age 30, you eat the perfect healthy diet and maintain a healthy weight, in the future, you will gain weight on that same healthy diet.

What can you do? You can either eat less and less as you age, or you can maintain and hopefully gain a little muscle as you age. Resistance training is now known to be very important at all ages. You don't need to become a hardcore bodybuilder; you just need to do enough to maintain what you have. Isn't this a good reason be active?

NUTRITION

THE FIRST PILLAR OF LIFE-LONG SUCCESSFUL FAT LOSS

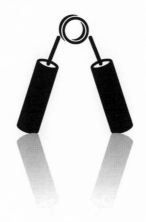

Chapter 16

If you think you can or you can't you are right." -Henry Ford

EVERYTHING YOU WANTED TO KNOW ABOUT MACRONUTRIENTS

THERE ARE THREE MAIN MACRONUTRIENTS in foods—fats, carbohydrates and protein. Remember when fat was bad for you in the 80's and 90's and people stopped eating eggs and beef? Then carbohydrates became evil a little bit later and everyone stopped eating bread and rice. Now, too much protein might cause kidney damage ... The reality is that you need all three to be healthy.

Most mainstream diets vary the ratios of these basic macronutrients. As well, if you look at most of the popular diets over time, they all seem to eat the same basic foods.

Here is a quick summary of what you need to know:

1. Carbohydrates

This is your body's main source of energy. Carbs are found in foods such as fruits, vegetables, breads, pastas, and rice. If you eat too many carbs, they will get stored as body fat. There are two types of carbohydrates: simple and complex. Simple carbs have a high sugar content and are absorbed by the body very quickly. Most "sinful" foods have a high percentage of simple carbs, but some healthy foods such as fruit are also in this category. These foods cause a huge spike in the amount of insulin your body releases. This type of carb is absorbed very quickly, but you are hungry soon after.

> Most "sinful" foods have a high percentage of simple carbs.

The body absorbs complex carbs slowly. There is not a large insulin spike after eating, and you will remain fuller much longer than if you had eaten simple carbs. The likelihood of complex carbs being stored as fat is much lower as well. Examples of complex carbs are multi grain breads and pastas, potatoes, yams, oatmeal, and most vegetables.

2. Protein

This is what your body is really made of. Every tissue in your body consists of proteins. Everything from your muscles and organs, to your skin, fingernails and hair.

The "fat phobia" of the 80's and 90's is probably the single greatest reason that the average person is fatter today.

Protein is found in all meats, eggs, milk, vegetables, beans, grains and legumes. Proteins are made up of amino acids. Your body can make 11 of the 20 essential amino acids. The rest of them, you must eat.

Most animal sources of protein are "complete" sources because they have all of the amino acids present in them. Vegetable sources of protein are "incomplete" and are missing various amino acids. If you are a vegetarian, you need to eat a variety of vegetables so that the combination of them will give you all of the amino acids that your body needs.

Just like carbohydrates, excess protein can be converted to fat.

3. Fats

All cells in your body contain some level of fat. Fats lubricate your joints and many of your hormones come from fats. Dry skin can be a symptom of not ingesting enough fat. It is vital that you do eat some fat in your diet.

The "fat phobia" of the 80's and 90's is probably the single greatest reason that the average person is fatter today. Thousands of products came to market that proclaimed to be "fat free" or low in fat. The problem with most of these products is that they had the same or even more calories than their original. The fat tended to be replaced by sugar. In fact, 100% sugar is fat-free. People felt that they had a license to eat as much as they wanted of low-fat food. They thought that they were eating healthy and moderately, but in reality the average person continued to gain more fat.

There are two types of fats

Saturated Fat—The Bad One You can spot most saturated fats just by looking at them. If it is solid at room temperature, it is probably saturated. It generally comes from animal sources and is found in foods such as butter, egg yolks, cheese, shortening and meat fat. This type of fat is linked to an increase in cholesterol, which can be a contributing factor in heart disease.

Unsaturated Fat—The Good One This type of fat is generally liquid at room temperature. This type of fat actually helps to lower your cholesterol! It is found in foods such as fish, walnuts, peanuts, safflower and sunflower oil and natural peanut butter.

There are some fats that your body cannot produce on its own. These are known as essential fatty acids (EFAs) and are found in most foods that have unsaturated fat in them. You may have heard the terms omega 6 or omega 3. These are two examples of EFAs that you can find as supplements in a health food store.

The Best Foods to Eat

Here are some examples of the best foods in each category.

Carbohydrates
The thing you need to watch out for here are refined carbohydrates. Refined carbs are generally white and are found in processed foods such as cookies, crackers, and white breads. Stick to things such as oatmeal, 100% whole wheat bread, whole-wheat pastas, brown rice, potatoes, yams, beans, lentils, etc. Just like your mother always used to tell you, you can never eat enough fruits and vegetables.

Protein
Not all sources of protein are of the same quality. Generally, if you choose animal based sources of protein, they will be complete proteins with all of the necessary amino acids. While a reasonable amount of fat is not bad for you, choose lean proteins. Examples of good sources are: chicken breast, turkey breast, fish, lean pork, lean red meat, fresh ham, eggs (limited number of yolks), milk (non-fat) and cottage cheese.

Fats
The worst thing that you can eat is any fried food or any product that contains "hydrogenated" or "partially hydro-genated" oils in the ingredients. Consuming saturated fats from red meat and egg yolks should be reduced, but not completely avoided. Some of the best fats are: flax seeds/oil, sunflower seeds/oil, fish oil (capsules or from fish), raw nuts, olive oil, avocados and natural peanut butter.

The worst thing that you can eat is any fried food or any product that contains "hydrogenated" or "partially hydrogenated" oils in the ingredients.

How much should you eat from each category?

This is the real difference between most diets.

High-carbohydrate diets

There were many popular diets in the last few decades that fell into this category. One of the best examples is the Pritikin diet. It was very similar to a vegetarian diet. In this diet, you eat 70% carbs, 20% protein, and 10% fat.

Low-carbohydrate diets

Many of today's most popular diets such as the Atkins, Sugar Busters, and the Zone limit that amount of carbohydrate you can eat. You may end up eating ratios such as 10% carbs, 55% protein and 35% fat.

A more reasonable approach

Everyone has a different body and a different metabolism. Some people get intense headaches, weakness and bad breath on low carb diets, while others have none of these side effects. Likewise, many people find that they are constantly hungry on high carb diets and never lose their cravings for a good steak, while a vegetarian may be the complete opposite. Instead of following the dogma of any specific diet, we suggest this approach.

Start with a basic diet of around 50% carbs, 30% protein and 20% Fat. choose to eat an amount of calories that is moderately below what you need to maintain your weight. Stay on this diet for a few weeks and see how you feel. If you feel awesome, don't change anything. As long as you have a moderate calorie deficit every day, you will lose weight.

If you want to experiment how you will feel eating more protein for example, you can increase your protein by 10% and lower your carbs by 10%. Continue to eat the same level of calories as you did before and again see how you feel a few weeks later.

Continue to adjust your ratios, until you find the optimal ratio for your body. The goal here is to experiment and learn what works for you. It is much easier to stick to a nutrition plan that works for your body and allows you to eat more of the foods that you enjoy. Remember, you are eating for a lifestyle change, not just for a temporary goal.

LISTENER QUESTIONS

Q Why should you eat more than three meals per day?

A If you search the Internet for tips for losing weight, eating multiple meals per day is a standard tip that you will find in almost every list. The advice will suggest to eat five or six small meals per day, or three meals with a few snacks.

This was not always the case. When Jeff was studying Physical Education in University, his textbooks were written in the mid-'80s and this was not stressed. The standard advice was to eat three square meals per day with perhaps one snack. In the mid-'90s, the evidence for the benefits of eating multiple meals each day grew to the point that it became the consensus. The benefits of eating often came from multiple areas of interest such as diabetes management relating to Insulin regulation, metabolism, and weight loss studies.

Eating five or six meals per day or three meals and a few snacks per day, is a recommendation from The American College of Sports Nutrition, Web MD, The Mayo Clinic, and the National Institutes of Health, just to name a few. There are people who disagree with this, but there is never 100% agreement on any health-related topic. If there was ever agreement on the perfect diet for instance, there would only be one diet book at the bookstore. There are literally thousands of diet books on the market today.

The main benefit of eating multiple meals throughout the day is that it speeds up your metabolism. The simplest way to tell if you metabolism is slow, is to rate your hunger in the morning. If you are hungry for breakfast, your metabolism is fired up. If you normally skip breakfast and don't get hungry until late afternoon, your metabolism is moving at a crawl. It is a myth that you only lose weight when you are hungry. You will lose weight over a 24-hour period based on the number of calories that you consume. There is no need to be hungry to lose weight if you only moderately reduce your calories.

> The main benefit of eating multiple meals throughout the day is that it speeds up your metabolism.

Japanese sumo wrestlers figured this out hundreds of years ago. A sumo wrestler only eats two large meals per day. Most people think that sumo wrestlers eat all day long, but they don't. They have found that one of the most effective ways to gain weight is to eat less often.

A second benefit is that if you eat multiple meals throughout the day, with lean protein and complex carbohydrates, this will help to regulate your insulin levels. It is also a myth that people will get large insulin spikes if they eat this often. Large insulin spikes occur when a person has overeaten and/or is eating processed foods full of simple carbohydrates and sugar. This is standard medical advice for management of type 2 diabetes. It is also a recommendation for people who are at high risk of developing type 2 diabetes.

A third benefit is that eating multiple meals per day enhances your athletic performance and recovery from physical activity. If you eat every three hours, you will never have low energy for any type of physical activity. You could go to the gym or go for a run at any time of the day and not feel lethargic. After your workout, nutrition is extremely important for recovery and repair of your muscles.

If you are concerned with keeping the muscle that you already have while reducing fat or gaining muscle mass, the key macronutrient that you need is protein. However, protein only stays in your system for about three hours before it is depleted. If you eat every three hours, your body will be repairing and recovering to its best ability all day long.

A final benefit is an important one for those seeking to lose fat. The more often you eat, the less hungry you will be. If you do get hungry, you probably only have an hour to wait before your next meal or snack. Compare this to eating a salad for lunch and then waiting six hours for dinner.

Some final advice is to make sure that with every meal you have some lean protein and complex carbohydrates. For example, a breakfast could have some eggs with a bowl of oatmeal, a lunch could have a chicken salad, and a dinner could have chicken, rice and vegetables. The goal is to eat the most food that you can, the most often, never feel hungry and lose fat at the same time. Eating mainly unprocessed foods will allow you to eat a much larger volume of food and feel fuller longer. One final word, is that no matter how many times you eat during the day, the total number of calories still must be under your maintenance level to lose fat.

Chapter 17

*"In eating, a third of the stomach should be filled with food,
a third with drink and the rest left empty." —Talmud*

THE FOOD ALL-STARS

WE ARE NOT GOING TO tell you what you can and cannot eat. Each person's tastes are different. If we did tell you exactly what to eat, the idea of lifestyle change would be thrown out the window. We would then be advocating just another diet. We do have some food suggestions to help in your fat loss.

The Fat 2 Fit Food All-Stars is a guideline, which ranks the best foods to the worst foods, but we leave it to you to decide. If you only ate from Five and Four-Star foods, you would have a near-perfect diet!

FIVE-STAR FOODS—PERFECT, EAT ANY TIME

Apples, with skin	Egg whites	Peas
Artichokes	Endive	Peppers
Arugula	Fish, cold water	Plantains
Asparagus	(salmon, mackerel,	Prunes
Avocados	sardines)	Radishes
Beans	Fish, freshwater	Raspberries
Beets	Flaxseed	Refried beans, nonfat
Bok choy	Garlic, fresh	Rice, brown
Boysenberries	Granola, raw, no sugar	Salsa, natural, no sugar
Bran	Hemp seed	Seitan
Broccoli	Kale	Spinach
Broccoli sprouts	Lettuce, romaine,	Squash
Brussels sprouts	green or red leaf	Strawberries
Cabbage	Milk, nonfat	Sweet potatoes
Carrots	Milk, soy	Tea, green or black
Cauliflower	Muesli, raw, no sugar	Tempeh
Celery	Mushrooms	Tofu
Cereal, whole grain	Mustard	Tomato sauce, no sugar
Chard	Nectarines	Tomatoes
Cherries	Oatmeal	Vinegar
Citrus fruits	Olive oil	Water
Collard greens	Olives	Yams
Cottage cheese, nonfat	Onions	Yogurt, nonfat, no sugar
Cucumbers	Pears, with skin	

FOUR-STAR FOODS—ALMOST PERFECT, HAVE YOUR FILL

Apples, skinless
Bananas
Blueberries
Bread, whole grain
Cantaloupe
Cheese, nonfat
Chicken, skinless white
    meat
Coffee, black or
    cappuccino with
    nonfat milk
Corn
Cottage cheese,
    low-fat
Cream cheese, nonfat
Duck, free-range
Eggplant
Fish, farmed

Granola or energy bar
Grapes
Hummus
Juice, fresh-squeezed
    with pulp, no sugar
Kiwifruit
Mangoes
Meal replacement
    bar
Melon, honeydew
Milk, 1%
Nuts, raw
Ostrich
Pancakes, buckwheat
Papayas
Peaches
Pineapple
Plums

Raisins
Ricotta cheese, nonfat
Soy nuts
Soy sauce
Squid
String beans
Sunflower seeds
Tortillas,
    whole wheat
Turkey breast
Vegetable juice
Veggie burger
Venison, free-range
Watermelon
Yogurt, no sugar
Zucchini

THREE-STAR FOODS—EAT SPARINGLY

A1 Steak Sauce
Angel food cake
Applesauce
Bagels
Beef, eye of round
Beef, London
Beef, top round
Canola oil
Cheese, low-fat
Chicken, dark meat
Chicken sandwich, broiled
Chicken taco, baked
Clams
Coffee, cappuccino with
    whole milk
Crab
Cream cheese, low-fat
Eggs, whole

French fries, baked
Fruit, dried
Graham crackers
Granola
Honey
Jam or marmalade
Jerky, turkey
Juice, from concentrate
Ketchup
Lamb, lean
Lettuce, iceberg
Lobster
Mayonnaise
Milk, 2%
Muesli
Oatmeal, flavored
Oysters
Pancakes

Pasta, plain
Peanut butter, raw
Popcorn, plain
Pork tenderloin
Potatoes, baked or
    boiled
Pretzels
Refried beans,
    low-fat
Rice cakes
Rice, white
Sauerkraut
Soup, canned broth
Steak, lean
Sweet-and-sour sauce
Veal cutlet
Wine, red
Yogurt, frozen, nonfat

TWO STAR FOODS—ONCE IN A WHILE

Animal crackers
Beef, filet mignon
Beef, lean ground
Beef, sirloin
Beef Stroganoff
Beer
Bread, refined flour
Buffalo
Butter
Caesar salad, with chicken
Canadian bacon
Cheese (including bleu
   & goat)
Chili
Chinese food
Chips, low-fat, baked
Coconut Coffee, iced
   mocha latte with
   nonfat milk
Coffee, latte with
   whole milk
Coffee cake

Crackers
Grilled cheese sandwich
Ham
Hot dogs, turkey
Ice cream, sugar-free
   or fat-free
Jell-O
Juice, sweetened
Lamb chops
Lasagna, with meat
Macaroni & cheese
Margarine
Meat loaf
Mexican food
Milk, whole
Muffins
Nuts, salted or roasted
Peanut butter, not raw
Pepper, stuffed
Pizza, meatless or
   Hawaiian style
Popcorn, with salt & butter

Pork chop
Potato salad or
   macaroni salad
Pudding, with low-fat milk
Reuben sandwich
Sherbet
Shrimp
Sloppy Joe, lean beef
   or turkey
Soft drinks, diet
Soup, canned creamy
Spaghetti, with meatballs
Sub sandwich
Taco salad, with chicken
Tortilla, refined flour or
   corn
Tuna salad or chicken
   salad
Vegetable oil
Wine, white
Yogurt, frozen

ONE STAR FOODS—SPECIAL OCCASIONS ONLY

Alcohol, hard liquor
Bacon
Baked beans
Beef, ground, regular
Beef taco, fried
Breakfast sandwich,
   fast food
Cakes
Candy
Cereal, sugared
Chicken a la King
Chicken, buffalo wings
   or nuggets
Chicken or fish
   sandwich, fried
Chips, potato or corn
Chocolate

Cinnamon bun
Coffee, mocha, macchiato,
   ice blended, frappé,
   triple caramel
   vanilla buzz bomb, etc.
Cookies
Cream cheese
Creamed veggies
Creamer, nondairy
Doughnuts
French fries
Gravy
Hamburger, fast food
Hot dogs
Ice cream
Jerky, beef, pork, or
   venison

Juice, sugar added
Lobster Newburg
Nachos
Onion rings
Pastries
Pies
Potato skins, fried
Potatoes, fried
Potpie
Refried beans,
   with lard
Salad dressing, creamy
Sausage
Soft drinks, sugared
Tater tots
Toaster pastries

LISTENER QUESTIONS

Q Is a calorie from junk food the same as a calorie from healthy food? Is it all a numbers game of calories in versus calories out, or do the type of calories (fat, protein and carbs) count too?

A Technically, a calorie is the amount of heat energy needed to raise one gram of water one degree Celsius. In the scientific sense of energy production, a calorie is just a calorie, but it doesn't hold true for humans.

An Olympic athlete may eat 3000 calories per day. They could probably eat 10 candy bars and drink two sodas every day to maintain their weight. Does anybody really think that their bodies would be able to continue to perform at the same level or look the same by eating this diet? Of course not. After eating a poor diet, they would feel horrible compared to how they feel when in top shape.

People who regularly eat this much junk food do feel horrible all the time, but they may not know it is from the food they eat.

People who regularly eat this much junk food do feel horrible all the time, but they may not know it is from the food they eat. They think that feeling tired and sluggish is normal.

It is true that if you are looking to lose fat, you need to eat fewer calories than you burn. But all calories are not created equal. Some calories will be more satisfying for your hunger, be more nutritious, burn more calories during digestion, and simply be more healthy.

Empty calories are calories which provide no nutritional value to a person. They provide no minerals, vitamins, fiber or anything else that one would consider to be healthy. An example would be sugary sodas or candy. They may taste good, but they will only have a minimal impact on your hunger. Since they are extremely processed foods, your body will convert them into sugar almost instantly. Because there will be such a quick spike of sugar in your bloodstream, your body's insulin will quickly convert it to storage as fat. Soon after, you will be hungry again.

When many people start eating a well-balanced diet and reduce their calories to lose fat, they find that they actually start eating much more food. The volume of food that you can eat when you are eating mainly unprocessed foods is much larger than the equivalent amount of junk food. For example, a Girl Guides cookie has 75 calories. You could eat three cookies or eat a turkey sandwich with lettuce, tomato, and sprouts. Many people will have no difficulty eating nine cookies, but eating three sandwiches is much different. The speed that your body digests food will make a big difference on your hunger. Junk foods take very little energy or effort from your body to digest. You can think of processed and junk foods to be partially "pre-digested" for you. When you eat complex carbohydrates such as vegetables, whole grain breads and pastas, potatoes or oatmeal, they digest very slowly and will leave you satisfied much longer. When you eat lean proteins such as eggs, meats and dairy, your body has to do a lot of work to break all of those chemical bonds in the food while digesting it. In fact, a portion of the calories in protein doesn't really count, because your body burns calories just to digest the protein. A chicken breast may contain 100 calories, but your body may take 20 calories of energy to digest the chicken breast, and that will leave you with 80 "net calories."

In our opinion, the ultimate goal of a dieter is to eat the most amount of great tasting food, feel satisfied, and never be hungry while you are losing fat or maintaining a healthy weight. This simply can't be done while eating calorically dense junk food.

Chapter 18

"Sure, it makes you happy in the short term, but it makes your fat happy in the long term." —Jeff Ainslie

THE GLYCEMIC INDEX

THE GLYCEMIC INDEX WAS INTRODUCED 30 years ago and is a measure of the effects of carbohydrates on blood glucose levels. The original purpose of the glycemic index was to determine the speed at which carbohydrates are broken down during digestion. Carbohydrates that break down rapidly and flood glucose into the bloodstream are considered high-glycemic foods and are not recommended to be eaten by people with diabetes. Carbohydrates that are broken down slowly and do not cause a glucose spike in the bloodstream are low-glycemic foods.

Here is a list of some high-glycemic foods. Most of these foods are also considered simple carbohydrates.

HIGH-GLYCEMIC FOODS

FRUITS
Most dried fruits
Bananas (ripe)
Papayas

BEVERAGES
Soft drinks & sport
  drinks (added sugars)
Carrot juice

SWEETENERS
Corn syrup solids
Sucrose (table sugar)
Glucose & glucose
  polymers (malto-
  dextrin-based drinks)
Honey
Maltose
High-fructose corn syrup
Barley malt

VEGETABLES
Parsnips
Potato (baked)
Cooked carrots
French fries
Yams
Sweet corn
Potato chips

DAIRY
Ice cream

GRAINS
White bread
Whole wheat bread
French bread
Bagels
Cold cereal
Breakfast cereals (refined
  with added sugar)

GRAINS CONTINUED
Corn chips
Cornflakes
Rice cakes
Crackers & crispbread
Doughnuts
Hamburger &
  hotdog buns
White rice
Muffins (due to the
  processed flour)
Pancakes
Puffed rice or wheat
Pretzels
Shredded wheat
Toaster waffles

Does this mean that you should always avoid high-glycemic index foods? Not necessarily. The ones that are low in nutrition and high in calories you should always avoid such as soft drinks and white bread. There are times that you might want a spike in your glucose and energy levels, such as right before you do resistance training or an intense activity. That doesn't mean that you have to eat something sugary though. Eating a banana will suffice most of the time.

On the other end of the glycemic index spectrum, carbohydrates that break down slowly, releasing glucose gradually into the blood, have a low glycemic index. You can see how this would be beneficial to those individuals with diabetes who are insulin resistant.

Here is a list of several low-glycemic foods. About half of these foods are considered complex carbohydrates, but there are several fruits that are considered simple carbohydrates.

LOW-GLYCEMIC FOODS

FRUITS
All berries
Cherries
Apples
Oranges
Peaches
Apricots
Plums
Grapefruit
Pears

NUTS AND SEEDS
Almonds, Walnuts
Peanuts
Flaxseeds
Pumpkin seeds
Sunflower seeds

SWEETENERS
Stevia
FOS (frycto-oligo-
    saccharides)

VEGETABLES
Artichokes
Asparagus
Black-eyed peas
Split peas
Bulgur
Azuki beans
Butter beans
Black beans
Garbanzo beans
Celery
All lettuces
Navy beans
Peppers
Soybeans
Tomatoes
Onions

GRAINS
All bran cereals
Oatmeal/Oat bran
Whole grain pastas
Barley

BEVERAGES
Fresh vegetable juice
Tomato juice
Green tea
Water

DAIRY
Organic milk
Organic plain yogurt (no
    added sugar)
Low-fat cottage cheese

Can following a low-glycemic diet help you lose weight? Maybe. If you are eating foods that have a low or high glycemic index **and** you are in a calorie deficit, you will lose weight. If you have diabetes or have several risk factors that may lead to diabetes, eating mainly low-glycemic foods is well advised.

Low-glycemic foods are not your weight loss savior, but if you take a look at the foods that are on the low glycemic list, you'll notice that they are foods that anyone would consider "healthy foods." The foods on the high glycemic list are more processed, easily digestible foods and not necessarily whole foods.

By eating mainly healthy unprocessed foods, you will be eating mainly low-glycemic foods.

If you look at the big picture of weight loss, the most important thing is to get the other 90% of healthy eating and nutrition down first before spending a lot of time being overly concerned about the glycemic index. By eating mainly healthy unprocessed foods, you will be eating mainly low-glycemic foods.

LISTENER QUESTIONS

Q Should you eat a snack even if you are not hungry?

A The question should really be "Why I am not hungry after three or four hours?" The sign of a slow metabolism is the lack of hunger. Many people who skip breakfast are not hungry until lunchtime or mid-afternoon. Some people go 18 hours without eating and without hunger.

These people have adapted their metabolism to be able to go long durations without nourishment, but they have also adapted their bodies to be fat storing machines. When they do eat, a larger percentage of those calories are not stored as glycogen in their cells, they are converted to fat for long-term storage. The way that your body prepares for a regular 18 hour fast is to store future energy needs as fat.

The sign of a slow metabolism is the lack of hunger.

We believe that the best fat loss program is one where you actually feel guilty to be losing weight because you are always eating and never feel hungry! Don't expect to lose five pounds per week, but expect to lose a regular amount of fat every week.

Keep in mind, it is important that you are not eating above your calorie goals during the entire day regardless of how many meals and snacks you eat.

Eating often is a strategy to speed up your metabolism. The faster your metabolism, the more food you can eat, and the faster you will lose fat. Think of eating often as part of your weight loss strategy. Being hungry isn't a sign that you are losing fat, it is a sign of short term deprivation.

Here are some suggestions to apply this concept.

1. **Eat mainly clean and healthy foods.** Reduce processed foods as much as possible. By doing this, you simply get to eat a much larger volume of food. Eating a meal with a lean chicken breast, some brown or basmati rice and a pile of veggies will take you 10 or 15 minutes to eat. That will be much more healthy and satisfying than eating one of those "health" bars that you can eat in three bites.

2. **Eat a lean protein with every meal.** Research has shown that protein keeps you fuller longer, and therefore reduces hunger. Protein is digested slowly as your body works to break apart all of those amino acid bonds, and those amino acids help your body to recover from exercise.

3. **Nothing is ever set in stone.** Based on your results, adjust your eating plan. If you find that you aren't losing fat, reduce your calories a little more. If you find that you are hungry later at night, make your mid-morning snack a little smaller and your night time snack a little bigger.

Chapter 19

"A man may fall many times but he won't be a failure until he says someone pushed him." —*Elmer G. Letterman*

COOKING FOR WEIGHT LOSS

Ingredients

Whole, unprocessed foods are they key. If there is nutritional information on the side of your food, it is a processed food. In our "All-Star" food rankings, you would have a near-perfect diet if you only ate from our four- and five-star foods. These foods consist of fresh vegetables and fruits, non-fat dairy, fish, white meat chicken, whole grain bread, etc.

Fresh Versus Frozen Versus Canned

Obviously fresh is the best, but frozen vegetables are most times frozen right after harvest and will be the closest to fresh. Canned, with a few exceptions, will be your last choice. Often they are filled with extra sodium and other preservatives that keep them tasting better longer.

Portions

Cooking for weight loss is not all about the ingredients; it's also about the portion size. No matter what the quality of the ingredients are, eating too much of them will not support fat loss. Look at the recipe you're using to prepare meals from, and note the portion size and stick to that amount.

Preparation of Meat

Even the leanest cuts of meat still have fat, so many recipes advise us to trim all visible fat before cooking. To easily cut off the fat, put the meat in the freezer for up to 20 minutes. This should be just enough time for the fat to begin to harden. This makes it much easier to trim. Also, partially freezing beef, lamb or pork makes it much easier to slice the meat thinly for stir-fries or salads.

When preparing chicken, cut off the skin. Let's compare a 4 oz. portion of chicken with and without the skin. Chicken breast with skin is 188 calories, 49 percent from fat. It has 10.5 grams of total fat, and 3 grams of saturated fat. Meanwhile, skinless chicken breast is 118 calories, with 11 percent of calories from fat. It contains just 1.4 grams of total fat and 0.4 grams of saturated fat.

Baking is by far one of the best ways to prepare foods with weight loss in mind. You can marinate with a liquid such as lemon juice or just leave the food as is. Be sure to keep your dish covered either with the lid or with tin foil to seal in moisture. From poultry, to fish, to veggies like squash and potatoes, baking is the perfect cooking method. Be careful not to spoil your healthy, baked items by putting fat filled condiments on the finished product.

Baking is by far one of the best ways to prepare foods with weight loss in mind.

Boiling is a great way to cook for saving fat and calories, but there is some nutrient loss in vegetables when they're boiled directly in water. To prevent nutrient loss, boil veggies such as potatoes in their skins, choose boil-in-bag varieties or steam them.

Broiling, cooking under direct heat, is nearly as ideal as baking, but don't be tempted to add butter, wine or oil; choose fruit juice, broth or just plain old water instead if you are making a sauce. Broiling is an ideal cooking method for meats and fish.

Microwave cooking is also an ideal preparation method for weight loss. You can buy a microwave steamer that allows vegetables to be steamed in the microwave or you can boil veggies in water. Steaming is preferable, because of the nutrient loss mentioned above. If you are pinched for time, in the supermarket there are now fresh, steam in the bag, microwave vegetables. These vegetables are ready in five minutes, but be careful not to get the version with the cheesy butter sauce.

Experiment with herbs and spices to add a variety of flavors to make your meals more enjoyable.

Non-stick cookware is the preferred choice when cooking for weight loss. Avoid adding tablespoons of canola or olive oil to get food to not stick. If you do add a small amount of oil to your pan, here is a tip from the Frugal Gourmet, "Hot pan, cold oil, food won't stick." Alternatively, you can use a spray on oil in either canola or olive oil. You get the benefits of the oil while greatly reducing the amount that you use.

Here are a few substitution suggestions that you can make in other areas of the kitchen.

- Choose Canadian bacon or turkey bacon instead of regular bacon to add pizazz to those turkey sandwiches.
- Use one egg and two egg whites per person in your favorite egg dishes or cakes, or cut fat and cholesterol completely by using egg substitute.
- Use fat-free chicken broth or fat-free milk in mashed potatoes, soups, gravies and stews.
- Try fat-free evaporated milk in creamy soups and casseroles instead of heavy cream.
- Substitute reduced fat cheeses for full-fat ones, and cut the amount you use.
- Choose reduced-fat sour cream or yogurt instead of full-fat versions for stews, dips, spreads, and dressings.
- Use reduced-fat or fat-free cream cheese instead of the regular version for cheesecakes when you just have to have a dessert.

As a final thought, you don't have to eat bland foods in order to lose fat. Feel free to experiment with herbs and spices to add a variety of flavors to make your meals more enjoyable.

LISTENER QUESTIONS

Q How do I figure out the calories in food and recipes that I make myself?

A There are five common ways that our listeners tell us they determine this:

1. **Take all of the individual ingredients and add up their approximate calories.** You also need to include anything used in the preparation such as butter, oils etc. Then you divide the total calories by the approximate serving size.

2. **You can always use a store bought product label as your baseline estimate.** Usually the food that you make yourself will be lower calories, so if you use the store bought estimates, you will

most likely over-estimate the calories that you are eating. If you are worried about calories it is always better to over-estimate rather than under-estimate.

3. **If you want to be very precise, you can get the exact measurement of volume or weight of each ingredient, figure out the calories and then total them.** Then you can measure out how many servings are in the final product and divide the total calories by the number of servings you ended up with.

4. **There are now many programs for your Smartphone, which will do all of the work for you.** When looking for apps for your Smartphone, you will find ones that will track your calories by individual ingredient, restaurants, or recipes. There is even a program called "Foodscanner" which allows you to use the camera in your phone to take a picture of a UPC code. This will automatically pull up all of the nutritional information of the food product that you just scanned.

5. **There are now a few online recipe calculators.** When you enter in the ingredients of the recipe, the calculator will do all the rest for you. One of the best ones is over at Sparkpeople.com (http://recipes. sparkpeople.com/recipe-calculator.asp).

Chapter 20

"The dictionary is the only place success comes before work. Hard work is the price we must all pay for success." —Vince Lombardi

DECIPHERING NUTRITION LABELS

P ART OF MAKING GOOD FOOD choices is knowing what is in the food you eat. If you buy an apple, you know it's an apple. But how about applesauce? It's just apples, right? Maybe not. It's time to check the nutritional label and the ingredients.

Manufacturers are required to provide ingredient lists and nutrition fact labels on any packaged food. These labels are your tools in helping you make healthier food choices. Becoming knowledgeable about how to read these labels will help you to make better decisions about foods you buy and prepare.

The Ingredient List

The largest ingredient in the food is listed first followed by the remaining ingredients in decreasing quantity. When deciding which foods to buy based on the ingredient list, there are a couple rules of thumb. First, if you have never heard of the ingredient or can't pronounce it, there is a good chance that it's a chemical or other unnatural ingredient and should be avoided. The second rule is try to choose whole foods or foods that you recognize all or most of the ingredients.

A few things to avoid when looking at the ingredient list are excessive sugars, fats and oils. Its not always easy to spot them. Sugar could be hiding as sucrose, dextrose, fructose, corn syrup, high fructose corn syrup, molasses, honey or bleached flour. Bleached flour isn't a sugar, but it has very little nutritional value and as a result the body processes it like sugar. Fats could be hiding in ingredients such as coconut oil, cream, hydrogenated soy bean oil, hydrogenated vegetable oil, palm oil, palm kernel oil, partially hydrogenated soy bean oil or lard.

The Nutritional Label

Serving Size It tells you the recommended serving size of the food. This section of the label also tells you how many servings are in the package.

Calories This will list the total calories per serving. Here is the first "gotcha" when it comes to reading the nutritional label. When reading the label, make sure you look at how many servings are in the package. All too often a package may look like a single serving. In reality there could be three or four servings in just one package. If you don't read the serving size accurately you will be eating more than you planned on.

Calories from fat is adjacent to the total calories. Fat calories tells you how many calories of the food are specifically fat calories. Ideally, no more than 30% of your calories for the day should come from fat.

Nutrition Facts

Serving Size 1/2 cup (about 82g)
Servings Per Container 8

Amount Per Serving

Calories 200   Calories from Fat 130

	% Daily Value*
Total Fat 14g	**22%**
Saturated Fat 9g	**45%**
Trans Fat 0g	
Cholesterol 55mg	**18%**
Sodium 40 mg	**2%**
Total Carbohydrate 17g	**6%**
Dietary Fiber 1g	**4%**
Sugars 14g	
Protein 3g	

Vitamin A 10%   •   Vitamin C 0%

Calcium 10%   •   Iron 6%

*Percent Daily Values are based on a 2,000 calorie diet. Your daily values may be higher or lower depending on your calorie needs:

	Calories	2,000	2,500
Total Fat	Less than	65g	80g
Saturated Fat	Less than	20g	25g
Cholesterol	Less than	300mg	300mg
Sodium	Less than	2,400mg	2,400mg
Total Carbohydrate		300g	375g
Dietary Fiber		25g	30g

Calories per gram:
Fat 9 • Carbohydrate 4 • Protein 4

Fat Fat is next on the label. Total fat is represented and is broken down into saturated fat, trans fats, polyunsaturated fat and monounsaturated fat. Trans fats are the worst of the offenders and should be eliminated from your diet. Trans fats are the ones that fast food restaurants are trying to eliminate from their fryers.

Cholesterol Cholesterol should be no more than 300 mg. The cholesterol may not be broken down into good cholesterol (HDL) and bad cholesterol (LDL).

Sodium Your total sodium should be no more than 2400 mg. per day. Sodium can be problematic for those with hypertension.

The sodium and cholesterol numbers are based on a percentage of recommended daily value. The daily value, and this is the same information on every label, is based on a 2000 calorie/day diet and should be adjusted up or down based on how many calories you eat.

Carbohydrates The carbohydrates section gives you the total amount of carbohydrates in the food. Carbohydrates are further broken down into fiber and sugar. When comparing foods in the grocery store, try to pick foods higher in fiber content and lower in sugar content.

Here's another good tip. When looking at total carbohydrates, the closer the sugar gram value is to the total carbohydrate gram value, the worse that food is for you.

Protein Grams of protein are given. We suggest that you should eat lean protein with every meal. If the food you are eating doesn't contain protein, pair it with some other food that does.

The **Daily Values** portion of the label tells you how much the recommended daily allowance the food contains, again based on the 2000 calorie diet. Generally a value that is around 5% would be considered low and a value of 20% or higher is considered high.

The **Vitamins and Minerals** section lets you know the specific types and amounts of each that you are eating. You should try and consume 100% for all the required vitamins and minerals each day through food, if possible.

The last section on the label is the **Recommended Amounts**. This section provides the recommended daily amounts for each nutrient for a 2000-calorie and a 2500-calorie diet. The interesting thing here is there is no recommended amount for protein. The carbohydrate and fats are given along with cholesterol and sodium.

Here is an interesting thing that you can do with a nutrition label. Take the total number of calories and divide that into the total fat calories. Foods that have 15% or 20% of your RDA of fat are, quite often, entirely fat. For example, the serving size on a salad dressing may be only 5% of your RDA but can consist of 50 to 90% fat. You could be basically eating pure fat.

When you are trying to eat a certain percentage of your calories in protein, carbohydrates and fats, it's a better choice to choose foods that are themselves in the correct macro-nutrient ratios. While that's not always possible, if you're eating a food that is almost completely fat, it's harder to balance out with other things in your meal.

LISTENER QUESTIONS

Q Does water help you lose weight? Will drinking 8 to 10 8-ounce glasses of water help?

A Yes, drinking water will help you lose weight. One major study completed in 2008 found that "Absolute and relative increases in drinking water were associated with significant loss of body weight and fat over time, independent of covariates." This means that just by ingesting more water, those people lost more fat. As a note, water even did better when compared to non-caloric beverages.

So how much water do you really need? Many different studies over the years have produced varying recommendations, but in reality, your water needs depend on many factors, including your health, how active you are and where you live.

Some of the most common suggestions are:

1. **Replacement approach.** The average person urinates 6.5 cups per day and loses 4 cups per day through breathing. 20% of a person's water is usually contained in their foods, so the recommendation is to drink 8 cups of water per day.

2. **Dietary recommendations.** The Institute of Medicine suggests that men drink 13 cups of beverages per day, and women nine.

3. **The rule of thumb is "Drink eight 8-ounce glasses per day."** This recommendation seems to come from the Food and Nutrition Board of the National Research Council, which, way back in 1945, said that you should do this. But what seems to have been forgotten is that the report added "Most of this quantity is contained in prepared foods." Omit that, and it changes their recommendation quite considerably.

> It is always best to drink water over other beverages if you are concerned with accelerating your fat loss.

We recommend that if you drink enough fluid so that you rarely feel thirsty and produce colorless or slightly yellow urine, your fluid intake is probably adequate. It is always best to drink water over other beverages if you are concerned with accelerating your fat loss, and it is better to drink a little extra water in a day rather than drink too little.

Chapter 21

"The food you eat can be either the safest and most powerful form of medicine or the slowest form of poison." —Dr. Ann Wigmore

ARTIFICIAL SWEETENERS

IF YOU ARE LOOKING TO replace the sugar in your diet with a product like Splenda, Equal, Sweet'N Low or even stevia, this chapter is a must read. There's a lot of marketing hype behind these products, so it's understandable that there could be some misconceptions about them.

These artificial sweeteners are chemical compounds that were concocted by chemists in a lab. They are extremely popular because their sweetness is many times that of sucrose (which is ordinary table sugar). As a result of this sweetness, much less of the sweetener is required and the calorie contribution to the product its added to is often negligible. Here is the background on artificial sweeteners:

Splenda is generically known as sucralose. It's one of the newer artificial sweeteners on the market. It was approved by the FDA in 1998. It's 600 times sweeter than table sugar.

Equal is generically known as aspartame. It is also sold as NutraSweet. Aspartame was approved by the FDA in 1981. It's 200 times sweeter than table sugar.

Sweet'N Low's generic name is saccharin. This artificial sweetener has been around the longest. It was approved by the FDA in 1958. It's 300 times sweeter than table sugar.

These artificial sweeteners are three out of the five that are approved for use as a sweetener for food in the United States. The other two are neotame and acesulfame potassium. Neotame is extremely new. It was approved by the FDA in 2002 and is 8,000 times the sweetness of table sugar. Acesulfame potassium is 200 times as sweet as table sugar. We haven't heard of any products that use these artificial sweeteners yet.

How about **Stevia?** Stevia is not a synthetic sweetener. It is actually an herb that is native to Paraguay and is 250 times sweeter than table sugar. It is used as a sweetener in other countries, but in the United States it is considered a dietary supplement.

The FDA has established the maximum amount a person can consume of these sweeteners on a daily basis. It's called the Acceptable Daily Intake.

ARTIFICIAL SWEETENER	ADI	ESTIMATED ADI EQUIVALENT	OK FOR COOKING?
Aspartame (NutraSweet, Equal)	50 milligrams (mg) per kilogram (kg)	18 to 19 cans of diet cola	No
Saccharin (Sweet'N Low, SugarTwin)	5 mg per kg	9 to 12 packets of sweetener	Yes
Acesulfame K (Sunett, Sweet One)	15 mg per kg	30 to 32 cans of diet lemon-lime soda	Yes
Sucralose (Splenda)	5 mg per kg	6 cans of diet cola	Yes

Safety of Artificial Sweeteners

Artificial sweeteners are often the subject of stories, presented in the popular press and on the Internet, claiming that they cause a variety of health problems, including cancer. According to the National Cancer Institute, however, there is no scientific evidence that any of the artificial sweeteners approved for use in the United States cause cancer. Numerous studies have confirmed that artificial sweeteners are safe for the general population.

Aspartame does carry a cautionary note, however. It is not safe for people who have the rare hereditary disease phenylketonuria (PKU). Products that contain aspartame must carry a PKU warning on the label.

Still Empty Calories

Just removing sugar from cookies and chocolates doesn't make them low-calorie, low-fat foods. If you eat too many, you will still get more calories than you need, and you may not get enough nutritious foods. Unlike fruits, vegetables and whole grains, sugar-free soft drinks, candy and desserts often provide few—if any—beneficial nutrients.

Use artificial sweeteners sensibly. It's okay to substitute a diet soda for a regular soda, for example, but diet soda shouldn't be the only beverage you drink.

What do we suggest?

It is always best to eat the most natural unprocessed foods that you can find, so perhaps Stevia might be better if you don't want to eat any artificially created products. One of the main problems with our society right now is that most people have become accustomed to eating things that are either heavily spiced or overly-sweet. If you quickly change your diet to one that has no sweetness at all, you might have a tough time sticking to that eating program because you will start to crave sweetness. You never want to remove any single item from your diet for the rest of your life. Everything in moderation.

Alternative sweeteners are great at helping you transition into eating healthier.

These products are great at helping you transition into eating healthier if you use them sparingly and in reasonable amounts. If you are following our life long strategy of eating like the thinner person that you want to become, the use of artificial sweeteners may not be just for saving some calories. Think of biting into a fresh, sweet ear of corn on the cob. That is natural sweetness, but many people over time find corn bland because their tastes have changed to expect much more than what nature can provide. If adding in a little artificial sweetness will help you to eat more healthy real foods, then overall it can be a good thing.

LISTENER QUESTIONS

Q What is the best way to cook and freeze meals in advance?

A Planning meals in advance is one of the best strategies to aid in fat loss. When you plan your meals in advance and have the ingredients at home and ready to cook, you are less likely to eat whatever food is convenient and make poor choices.

Cooking and freezing meals for future use is also a good strategy. These meals are always ready to be reheated. When you have healthy meals ready to eat, there is no excuse to eat poorly. Don't have time to prepare a healthy lunch every morning? Just grab a homemade frozen lunch on the way out the door.

On the Fat 2 Fit Radio show, we advocate preparing many meals in advance. Jeff prepares as many as 35, or seven weeks of weekday lunches, at the same time. Every meal does not have to be identical, and many different meals can be prepared at the same time. In Jeff's case, spending three hours cooking large batches of food and then creating individual meals ensures that two months of lunches are ready. Because he doesn't take a frozen meal every day, those frozen lunches may last up to three months.

Frozen healthy meals: Isn't it nice to have and not need, than need and not have?
All that it takes is the freezer space and the desire to do so. The simple lunch that has been highlighted on the Fat 2 Fit Radio web site, is chicken, rice (basmati or brown) and mixed vegetables.

One out of three items is already frozen, the vegetables. The chicken is baked in the oven with spices of your choice. Once cooked it is diced or cut into the appropriate serving size per container. A portion of rice is then added to the container and the balance of the space in the container is filled with frozen vegetables. The containers that you fill can be stacked in your freezer. The only limiting factors are the size of your freezer and the number of storage containers you are willing to earmark for your future lunches/dinners.

The real expert in the correct procedures for freezing foods is the National Center for Home Food Preservation.
On their web page (http://www.uga.edu/nchfp/how/freeze.html) they highlight the best way to freeze many types of foods. Did you know that avocados are best frozen as puree? Did you know that you should blanch black-eyed peas two minutes before you freeze them?

All that information, and more, is available for your meal-freezing endeavors.

Chapter 22

*"Even though I overeat in private, excess poundage
is there for the world to see." —TOPS*

NEGATIVE CALORIE FOODS—FACT OR FICTION?

YOU MIGHT HAVE HEARD THIS one: It takes more calories to digest celery than you get from eating it. Most things that seem too good to be true usually are—except this one. This is fairly truthful. Here is the explanation.

Humans cannot digest the cellulose in plants, so vegetables and fruits with high cellulose content are not efficiently digested. Animals such as cows or horses can thrive by eating grass, but as humans we would starve.

All foods have calories in them. An 8-inch celery stalk has about six calories that we can digest. When you subtract the amount of energy that our body takes to digest the celery, the net caloric effect may turn out to be nothing at all. This is why celery has turned out to be a dieter's staple food.

By eating a sensible diet that includes several of the "negative calorie" foods, you can lower the net amount of calories that you are eating. As well, if you are eating a calorie reduced diet and are finding that you are not satisfied with the amount of food that you are eating, you can eat more of these "negative calorie" foods. This will add more bulk to your food, and this should help you feel a little fuller from your meals.

Keep in mind; in the same way that you can't survive on grass, you can't survive on just these foods alone. You still need to be eating other quality foods for the nutrients, minerals, vitamins and calories that your body needs.

Here is a list of some of the more common "negative calorie" foods

Vegetables Asparagus, beets, broccoli, cabbage (green), carrots, cauliflower, celery, chicory, chili peppers, cucumbers, endive, garlic, lettuce, onions, papayas, spinach, turnip, and zucchini.

Fruits Apples, cranberries, grapefruit, lemons, mangos, oranges, pineapple, raspberries, strawberries, and tangerines.

Should you count those calories in your daily caloric count? There are two camps here. One side says that you must count those calories and the other side says that it should be bonus food. We suggest the best approach might be to go somewhere in the middle. Many people find that counting half the calories a good way to encourage them to eat more of these healthy foods and still be accountable for all the food they are consuming.

LISTENER QUESTIONS

Q Is it true that drinking ice cold water will burn calories and help me lose weight?

A Studies have shown that drinking water will speed up a person's fat loss. Even when you compare water to no-calorie drinks, water is the best.

A person's body temperature wants to stay at 98.6° F or 37° C. The thought is that since your body will take energy to warm up the cold water, you will burn calories. The technical definition of a calorie is the energy required to raise 1 gram of water up one degree Celsius.

Since ice water is at zero degrees Celsius, it will need to be raised 37 degrees. There are 237 grams in an 8-ounce glass of water. When all of the math is done and you convert the number of calories into kilo-calories (this is how we really refer to calories in food), you will burn 8.75 calories heating up that 8-ounce glass of ice water in your belly.

So does drinking ice water help you lose weight? Yes, a very, very small amount. If you drink four hundred 8-ounce glasses of ice water, it may help you lose one pound.

On the flip-side, eating hot food or drinking hot beverages would also burn more calories, because you body needs to cool them down to your body temperature. If your body sweats, you are burning calories.

This is something that is technically true, but in the grand scheme of fat loss, it is the minutiae and not important. Don't let the minutiae distract you from your goals. Focus on the 95% part of weight loss, eating healthy with a reduction in calories, and increasing your exercise.

Chapter 23

"We are what we repeatedly do. Excellence, then, is not an act, but a habit." —*Aristotle*

TOP 7 NUTRITION STRATEGIES FOR SHEDDING FAT

PROPER NUTRITION IS THE KEY to overall health and especially fat loss. Keep in mind that you need to control your portion sizes to control your weight, but these strategies will turbo-charge your weight loss.

1. Prepare most of your meals in advance and have healthy snacks on hand.

If you have some healthy staple foods in the fridge, such as cooked turkey, chicken, and raw veggies, it is easy to stick to your eating plan. Don't get stuck without food which forces you to select bad choices such as fast food. If you prepare your own food, you can control how it is prepared, the quality, and the portion size. If you are hungry and are tempted to snack, make sure you have something healthy ready. Just because you had an extra snack doesn't mean that it has to be a disaster.

2. Try to eat every three hours.

If you don't have the time for five or six quality meals, have three meals and two or three snacks. This speeds up your metabolism. It keeps your blood sugar levels at a near constant level throughout the day and keeps you from being hungry. Eating small frequent meals fires up your fat burning furnace. Remember, Sumo wrestlers eat only one or two times per day. Their metabolisms greatly slow down between their meals making it easier for them to put on fat.

3. Do not eat until you are full.

By the time you realize you are full, you have already overeaten. A large meal will have excess calories that can be stored as fat. Get used to eating smaller meals, but more often.

4. Have a lean protein with every meal.

Protein is what your body is made of. It is used to build and repair your muscles, tissues, organs etc. It only stays in your blood stream for about three hours, so you need to eat it often. Another benefit of protein is that it takes more energy to digest than carbs or fat, so your net calories from eating protein are a little lower. Just make sure that you are eating lean proteins such as chicken breasts, white turkey, or egg whites.

5. Eat natural foods from Mother Nature, not a box.

Any processing of food reduces the quality of that food. Mother Nature does make it best. That is the easiest way to avoid things such as trans fats and excess sodium.

6. Do not drink your calories.

Eat an apple instead of apple juice. With an apple, you get more nutrients and fiber and less calories than drinking apple juice. Calories in liquids don't satisfy you like "real" food does. If you drink a sugary soft drink with a meal, you generally don't eat any less.

7. Give yourself one cheat meal per week.

If you are eating six quality meals per day, you are eating 42 meals per week. Having one meal "off" per week is good for your sanity and your social life. Just keep that meal reasonable, and don't let a cheat meal become a cheat day!

LISTENER QUESTIONS

Q How much bad stuff can I eat in a day? For example, how much chocolate can I enjoy guilt free?

A A "diet" tells you what you can and can't eat. This is why all "diets" fail in the long term. Our philosophy is to live the lifestyle of the thinner person that you want to become for the rest of your life, not go on a "diet."

We are not going to tell anybody what they can or can't eat or how much of anything they are allowed to eat. Our goal is to educate people about health and fitness so that they are capable of making the best choices. If we give strict guidelines about what we think people should eat on a daily basis, we would be falling into the trap of the rest of the diet industry. It is all about choices and moderation.

If you are on a strict diet, anything that you eat that is not in the diet plan will break the rules of that diet. We believe in the 90% rule. If you eat very healthy and exercise 90% of the time, you will do just fine and probably much better than average. When you deny yourself certain foods, you will only end up craving them more.

Jeff knows a person who eats one chocolate bar every single day. He eats one of the healthiest diets out there, full of fruit and vegetables, whole grains etc. and exercises almost every day. He loves chocolate and rewards himself with a little bit every day. Because he is a very active person, he eats somewhere in the range of 2800-3000 calories per day. One chocolate bar for him is less than 10% of his daily calories. His daily nutrition on the whole, is probably healthier than the average person's who never eats a chocolate bar. He rarely eats or drinks anything else with sugar in it, and he doesn't eat many processed foods. For him, this is his little reward that helps to keep him on track. If he never allowed himself this guilt-free treat, he many not be as successful as he is.

Two Final Points

1. Calories in versus calories out does work, but all calories are not created equal. Nutrition is extremely important to your health and how you feel on a daily basis.

2. As for saving up to eat some sinful foods, that is really up to you. You do have to keep in mind that you can't save up good nutrition. You can't only eat fruit and vegetables for every meal for two weeks and then eat junk for the rest of the year. What goes into your body comes out. If you put junk in, even if they are low calories, you will not have a healthy body. Feeling healthy and strong is just as important as looking healthy and strong.

Chapter 24

"It is never too late to be who you might have been."
—George Eliot

HOW TO BECOME A VEGETARIAN

THERE ARE MANY DIFFERENT INTERPRETATIONS of what it means to be a vegetarian. Here is the Wikipedia definition:

"Vegetarianism is the practice of following a plant-based diet including fruits, vegetables, cereal grains, nuts, and seeds, with or without dairy products and eggs. A vegetarian does not eat meat, including: red meat, game, poultry, fish, crustacea, shellfish, and products of animal slaughter such as animal-derived gelatin and rennet.

"There are a number of vegetarian diets. A lacto-vegetarian diet includes dairy products but excludes eggs, an ovo-vegetarian diet includes eggs but not dairy products, and a lacto-ovo vegetarian diet includes both eggs and dairy products. A vegan diet excludes all animal products, such as dairy products, eggs, and honey. Vegetarianism may be adopted for ethical, health, environmental, religious, political, cultural, aesthetic, economic, or other reasons."

To become a vegetarian is usually quite a lifestyle change for most people. We wanted to find out some tips and tricks that would help people to transition to a vegetarian lifestyle if they were intending to do so. We contacted Jennifer McCann who is a vegetarian and author of the *Vegan Lunch Box* series of cookbooks to ask her for advice.

Here are Jennifer's words of wisdom for new vegetarians.

I think the biggest **don't** is, "Don't assume that just because something is vegetarian or vegan it is better for you or even good for you." Potato chips and soda pop? Totally vegan. When I first went vegan years ago that's exactly how I ate—french fries, candy, etc. and hardly a vegetable in sight. Needless to say, I didn't feel too good after a while, and I certainly wasn't healthy. Avoid the temptation to fill the newly empty spots on your plate with foods made with lots of sugar and white flour, or with high-fat, deep fried foods.

I would say the biggest **do** is "Do start out by educating yourself as much as you can." There are a lot of wonderful books and websites out there on vegetarian and vegan nutrition and plant-based eating. I highly recommend *Becoming Vegetarian* and *Becoming Vegan* by B. Davis and V. Melina and the website veganhealth.org as good starting points to learn more about vegetarian nutrition.

Some people might disagree, but if you want to be healthy I would say the next **don't** is "Don't focus your new diet on fake meats." Nowadays you can find soy turkey slices, sausage, hot dogs, cheese, chicken nuggets, bacon, etc. to the point where you could continue eating exactly the way you did before, using all vegetarian replacements. When you replace the meat in your diet with fake meat, I don't think you're getting ahead nutritionally in the same way you would if you were replacing the old foods in your diet with whole plant foods. Fake meats are highly processed foods and are very high in sodium, and they also may keep you from branching out and experiencing new things.

That brings me to my next **do**: "Do focus every meal on whole plant foods." Whole plant foods like beans, vegetables, fruits, and whole grains are nutrient dense, rich in fiber, low in calorie, and high in disease-fighting phytochemicals. Best of all for those trying to lose weight, they are filling without being high in calorie. Other whole plant foods such as nuts, seeds, and avocado are not as low in calorie, but are nutrient dense and satisfying; daily servings in moderation will provide you with important healthy fats and help you feel full.

> Fake meats are highly processed foods and are very high in sodium, and they also may keep you from branching out and experiencing new things.

Sometimes a new vegetarian or vegan can start to focus on all the things they can't have anymore, and that can lead to feeling deprived. So **do** add new, healthy whole plant foods to replace every food you've given up. For example, shop for and try out new vegetables, grains, and beans; look through vegetarian and vegan cookbooks and try new recipes; visit ethnic restaurants and try out new cuisines. If you start focusing on what's new in your diet, you won't be focusing on what you can't have and feeling deprived.

Regarding supplements, **do** include a multivitamin that includes vitamin B12 and D to your daily diet, especially if you're switching to a vegan diet. You should also include daily sources of healthy fats, especially DHA and omega-3 fatty acids from vegetarian sources like flax seed and DHA algae. If you're vegan, make sure you're getting a good source of calcium, like calcium-fortified juices and non-dairy milks, dark leafy greens, okra, almonds, etc.

Of course a lot of people also worry about **protein**, but if you meet your daily calorie requirement by eating a wide variety of whole foods, you will probably be getting adequate protein without much effort. Good sources of protein in a vegan diet include beans and legumes, whole grains, soy foods such as tofu and tempeh, wheat gluten, peanut butter, nuts and seeds. Vegetarians, of course, also consume dairy products and eggs, two more good sources of protein. Whenever I feel like I need a little protein boost, I also add a mix of hemp, pea, and brown rice protein powder to a smoothie.

LISTENER QUESTIONS

Q Is it okay to get most of my protein from protein powders, shakes and supplements?

A Protein is an extremely important macronutrient. Protein contains amino acids, which are the building blocks of muscle. Protein helps people keep the muscle that they have, and is needed if you are trying to gain muscle. However, protein only stays in your system for about three hours, so that is one of the main reasons that we suggest that you eat often throughout the day. If there is no protein in your system, your body will not be repairing or building muscle as efficiently as when it is flooded with those amino acids.

To answer the question about whether protein powders can replace the lean protein portion of a meal, the answer is yes, but this would only be for convenience once in a while and should never be a major source of protein in your diet. There is always the scale of good, better and best. It is definitely not the best source, but it is always better than going with nothing.

There are four main reasons why lean protein, such as a chicken breast is better than protein powders, shakes and supplements.

1. **Protein powder does have calories.** Many people do not count those calories and that can end up sabotaging their fat loss. Many people will add an extra protein supplement to a smoothie, but that can add an extra 100 calories.

2. **Protein has the highest thermic effect.** The thermic effect of food is the amount of energy required to digest the food itself. It takes a lot of energy to digest a chicken breast. If you eat a 100-calorie chicken breast, your body may take 20 calories to digest it, and at the very end, your body only has 80 calories of it left. You can think of protein powder as being pre-digested. Because it is already highly processed, your body does not take any energy to digest it and break apart all of the chemical bonds.

3. **Real food has vitamins, minerals, fiber etc.** Protein powder is the ultimate processed food. Some powders add back in vitamins and other things, but it is still not as good as eating real food in its natural state.

4. **Satiety. Real food makes you feel full.** A thousand calories of protein powder has no impact on whether you feel hungry or not.

Chapter 25

"If people were as creative in coming up with solutions as they were in coming up with excuses, there would be a lot fewer problems in the world."—Tom Venuto

FAST FOOD

B ECAUSE OF ALL OF THE obligations and demands on people today, cooking a healthy meal at home is an activity that isn't as common as it once used to be. Due to lack of time or effort, fast food is a staple in many people's diets.

Here are some realities of fast food:

- Fast foods are not as healthy or nutritious as equivalent foods cooked at home.
- Fast foods contain higher levels of salt.
- Fast foods contain higher levels of calories than equivalents.
- Fast foods are mainly processed food products full of stabilizers, preservatives, flavor enhancers etc.

Eating fast food is never the best alternative. In reality, there will be situations where a person may have no other alternative than to eat fast food. Given that situation, a person can still make better choices with what is available.

Some guidelines that will help you make "better bad choices"

Be aware of the calories that you are eating. Most, if not all restaurants, have a nutritional guide posted or they will give you one upon request. If you frequent a particular fast food restaurant, know what items on the menu are the best for you and the number of calories that they contain. Limit yourself to those items. Just because you are in McDonald's doesn't mean you have to eat a Big Mac and a large fries. There are good choices at any restaurant that you visit.

On those rare occasions that you find yourself with no packed lunch and a restaurant without a nutritional guide, here are a couple guidelines to remember when ordering any item on the menu.

- Fried is bad, any other form of cooking is better.
- Chicken is better than beef, grilled instead of crispy.
- If a burger is the only choice, get it dry with lettuce and tomato.
- Choose a salad instead of fries when available.
- Get your kids the sliced apples or fruit cup instead of fries.
- Watch out for the extras and dressings on salads, get used to saying "Dressing on the side." Dressing can make a big difference:
    Caesar Pollo Salad, no dressing: 220 cals, 7 g. fat
    Caesar Pollo Salad, with dressing: 520 cals, 38 g. fat
- Get a salad that is made up of different greens, not just iceberg lettuce.
- Skip the soda and get a cup of water instead.

When most people see a fast food nutritional guide, they are often shocked when they learn the calories of their favorite foods. Legislation in different parts of the United States is being passed to compel fast food restaurants to put the calories and nutritional information right on the menu. Those laws are far from common right now. Until then, rely on educating yourself and not eating mindlessly when you find yourself unprepared.

LISTENER QUESTIONS

Q Is high fructose corn syrup really that bad?

A High-fructose corn syrup is a popular ingredient in many sodas, fruit-flavored drinks and other processed foods. It extends the shelf life of foods and is a replacement for sugar.

Milling corn to produce cornstarch produces high-fructose corn syrup. The cornstarch is then further processed to yield corn syrup, which is almost entirely glucose. In the final step, enzymes are added to change the glucose into fructose, which results in the syrup.

Food and drink manufacturers use it for several reasons. Consumers prefer its taste as it's sweeter than refined sugar, its syrupy consistency makes it easier to blend into soft drinks than refined sugar, and it's very inexpensive to produce. So inexpensive, in fact, that the National Soft Drink Association reported saving hundreds of millions of dollars by switching to high fructose corn syrup in the 1980s.

Many nutrition experts blame the increased consumption of high-fructose corn syrup for the growing obesity problem. There are current studies that show people put on more fat eating foods with high fructose corn syrup compared to food with sugar. One theory is that fructose is more readily converted to fat by your liver than is sucrose, increasing the levels of fat in your bloodstream.

In addition, animal studies have shown a link between increased consumption of high-fructose corn syrup and adverse health effects, such as diabetes and high cholesterol.

Unlike glucose, which stimulates the secretion of insulin, which transfers sugars to the body's cells, fructose does not stimulate insulin secretion. Furthermore, while glucose produces leptin, a hormone that helps regulate appetite and breakdown of fat storage, fructose does not produce leptin either. Thus, consuming high amounts of fructose found in corn syrup contributes to weight storage and overindulgence.

High fructose corn syrup originally comes from a natural source, but after all of the processing, all of nature's goodness is gone. Eating pure sugar is even healthier for you than consuming products with high fructose corn syrup.

Chapter 26

"The secret to staying young is to live honestly, eat slowly and lie about your age."
—Lucille Ball

OATMEAL RECIPES

O ATMEAL IS PROBABLY ONE OF the best things that you can eat as part of a healthy breakfast. It is low in calories and full of complex carbohydrates which keeps you fuller longer. Simple carbohydrates are digested very quickly and do not satisfy your hunger for very long. Foods such as donuts or pastries are examples of simple carbohydrate foods.

Over the years, as we have discussed the benefits of oatmeal, we have received many oatmeal recipes from our listeners. Here are three of the most popular oatmeal recipes:

Pre-packaged instant oatmeal is not very healthy. Here is how to make your own healthy version of instant oatmeal.

Instant Oatmeal

by Gail | makes eight packets

Ingredients
3 cups quick oats, salt, sugar (or sweetener)
8 zip sandwich bags

Process 1 cup of oats in a blender, 1/2 cup at a time, until it is as fine as flour.

In each sandwich bag measure 1/4 cup oats, 2 tablespoons oat flour, 1/4 teaspoon salt, 1 tablespoon sugar or equivalent sweetener

Directions
Mix a packet with 3/4 cup boiling water, stir, and let set 2 minutes.

Variations
Apple Cinnamon   Add 1/4 teaspoon cinnamon and 2 tablespoons chopped dried apples to each packet.

Cinnamon Spice	Add 1/4 teaspoon cinnamon and 1/8 teaspoon of nutmeg to each packet
Raisin Brown Sugar	Replace white sugar or sweetener with brown sugar or sweetener and add 1 tablespoon raisins to each packet.
Wheat germ	Add 2 tablespoons wheat germ to each packet.

One of Jeff's favorites comes from Tom Venuto, the fitness guru, and it's not just for regular oatmeal. This is the infamous oatmeal pancake recipe. These pancakes don't necessarily need to be refrigerated and are great for a snack as well as breakfast.

High Protein Oatmeal Pancakes

by Tom Venuto

Ingredients

1 cup Quaker Quick Oats or old-fashioned oatmeal
4 egg whites

1/2 apple, diced
1 scoop protein powder
1 tsp cinnamon

Directions

Put all ingredients together in a mixing bowl. Stir until the mixture has a semi-liquid pancake-batter-like consistency. Spray some non-stick spray on a frying pan and pour the mixture into the pan. Cook on medium heat. When one side is lightly browned and solid enough to flip, turn the pancake over with a spatula and cook the other side until lightly browned and firm.

Notes: For higher protein diets, add one scoop of vanilla protein powder (Designer Protein brand vanilla praline adds a nice flavor too). Wrap up your pancake in foil and take it to go, put it in the fridge for later use, or eat it hot! Oatmeal pancakes will stay fresh all day long without refrigeration.

Yield: 1 large pancake, 423 calories per pancake, 6 grams fat, 39.5 grams protein, 53.5 grams carbs

And finally, a listener made a comment on the web site and shared what has been the most popular searched for oatmeal item, breakfast oatmeal cookies. They are big and are a meal in themselves.

Oatmeal Breakfast Cookies

by Paxye | makes three servings

Ingredients

1 cup oats	1 tsp baking powder
1 cup skim milk powder	3 Tbsp whole wheat flour
1 Tbsp raisins	2 tsp brown sugar
1 Tbsp chocolate chips	1/4 tsp salt
1 cup apple sauce	1 tsp cinnamon

Directions

Preheat oven to 350°. Mix dry ingredients together (can be made in advance). Add applesauce and mix. Adjust if too dry or too wet. Make three mounds (they will be big and you can only fit two on a normal cookie sheet) and bake for 15-20 minutes until done.

350 calories per cookie, 3.2 grams fat, 4.2 grams fiber, 19.2 grams protein

EXERCISE

THE SECOND PILLAR OF LIFE-LONG SUCCESSFUL FAT LOSS

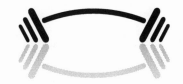

Chapter 27

"If you can't do great things, do small things in a great way. Don't wait for great opportunities. Seize common, everyday ones and make them great." —*Napoleon Hill*

THE IMPORTANCE OF EXERCISE

OUR BODIES ARE MEANT TO be active. Without exercise, our muscles atrophy and become weaker, our mental abilities deteriorate, and our life expectancy decreases. If you want to have a healthy, strong and lean body full of vitality and energy well into your old age, a lifestyle that includes exercise is a must.

Here are a few reasons to exercise:

- It improves your body shape.
- Provides more muscle definition.
- It helps alleviate varicose veins.
- Makes your clothes look better on you.
- It improves circulation and helps lower blood pressure.
- Strengthens your bones.
- Enhances oxygen transport throughout the body.
- Helps prevent heart disease.
- It decreases triglycerides in your blood.
- Increase your self confidence and your self-esteem.
- Reduces tension and stress.
- Helps alleviate depression.
- It enhances clarity of your mind.
- Increases your ability to problem solve.
- It helps you live longer.
- Helps you sleep better.
- Gives you more energy.
- Strengthens your immune system.
- It helps to ease or eliminate back problems and pain.
- It is a wonderful way to enjoy nature and the great outdoors.
- Improves endurance and stamina.
- Improves blood flow through out your body.
- It lowers your risk of death from cancer.

- Improves athletic performance.
- Increases your metabolic rate.

On episode #95 of Fat 2 Fit Radio, we listed these 25 reasons and also added another 100! We also asked our listeners why they want to become fit. Here is a sample of the reasons why they are exercising:

- To feel better physically.
- To be able to do more fun things.
- Peace of mind knowing I'm taking care of myself.
- To enjoy the way I look.
- In case of some sort of disaster, I will be able to help and not hinder.
- So I can sit on the floor and get up without grunting.
- To swing dance, and not feel sorry for the guy.
- To have regular bowels again.
- To keep up with my dog.
- So I can run away from bad guys!
- I hate the feeling when I sit down and I feel my stomach on my legs!
- I love the feeling when I've exercised and I'm eating well and I hit the scale and there's some loss. It feels like I'm in control, and I've got the discipline to reach my goals.
- I love when people see me and say, hey, you've lost some weight.
- I have found that I really enjoy running outside in the fresh air.
- I want to live a really long life and have many adventurers. Less pounds of fat means a healthy heart.
- I want to teach my kids healthy habits now so they don't spend a lifetime being overweight like I have.
- Sex with the hubby is better when my belly isn't flapping around!
- Shopping is considerably more fun when you step out of the "plus" section.
- I want to be viewed as an athlete.
- I have more energy now and can't wait to see what kind of energy I have when I reach my goal!
- My teeth feel cleaner since eating whole foods.
- More stamina in everything that I do.
- Compliments from friends/co-workers.
- Less prone to injury doing basic things—I used to strain my back on a regular basis, a couple or three times a year.

If you want to live the lifestyle of a thinner, healthier person, exercise is part of that lifestyle. Which of these reasons appeals the most to you?

LISTENER QUESTIONS

Q I am really confused about pre and post workout nutrition. There are so many conflicting theories about whether to eat before or after a workout and even more theories about what to eat, if you eat at all. So what and when should I be eating?

A If you are a professional athlete, bodybuilder or fitness model, every tiny advantage will help you. For the average person who wants to be well above average in fitness and health, and still have a regular lifestyle, the exact timing of nutrition isn't that important.

If your main goal is to lose weight in a reasonable manner, eating an overall healthy diet of five or six small meals, or three meals and two or three snacks throughout the day is all that you need to do. We always suggest that with every meal you have some lean protein like chicken or fish and healthy carbs like brown rice, fruit, veggies, oatmeal, etc. For an average person doing an average workout, you will do fine.

It is important that you don't work out when your body has low blood sugar. Without energy, it is hard to do a decent calorie-burning workout. If you are doing resistance training, not having enough energy will be the difference of getting those last few reps in—which is where all of the benefit of weight lifting happens.

After a good workout, your body will be craving protein to help recover from the workout and to repair all of those microscopic tears in your muscle fibers. Many bodybuilders will suggest that you drink a protein shake right after you work out. It is true that protein only stays in your system for about 3 hours, so by eating protein often, your body will always have the fuel it needs to repair itself.

As long as you are eating five or six meals per day, complete with a lean protein and "good" carbohydrates, you will be eating every three or four hours. In effect, you will be eating before and after each workout. If your concern is getting enough protein after your workout, you will be much farther ahead eating protein every three or four hours rather than getting a large protein spike from a shake right after training.

Q I am a student with a full-time job which makes me a super-busy person. Would it be better to get up and exercise first thing in the morning, or is it okay to try and get a quick cardio workout in the evening? I am more likely to do that than get up at 5 a.m. to work out, but I would be willing to if that would be more beneficial to my weight loss.

A The most important thing is that you work out at some point during the day. There is a debate over whether you burn more fat when you exercise first thing in the morning before you eat, but in reality, you lose weight over a 24-hour period based on your calorie balance during the whole day. Getting a workout in whenever you can, will not only burn calories and speed up your metabolism. It will also refresh your mind for your studies.

Many people work out late in the evening for a variety of reasons. Some wait until their children are put to bed, or until all of their commitments for the day are completed, or perhaps they want to avoid the crowds at their local gym. Some people find that doing a good workout right before bed helps them sleep, but some find that it keeps them up for hours.

The best workout is any workout, at any time.

Others work out very early in the morning. The main reason why people will wake up at 4:30 or 5 a.m. is because this may be the only time in the day that they can guarantee that they will always be free of commitments. Many people find that a good workout early in the morning wakes them up and they feel more prepared to take on the day. Others find that by getting up so early, they are exhausted and ready for bed by 8 p.m.!

Remember, if you are working out to improve your health, reduce your body fat, and sharpen your mind for school or work, the best workout is any workout, at any time.

Lastly, try to do the workout that is the most efficient for you and burns the most calories. If you use cardio equipment, your best bet would be an elliptical trainer, followed by a stair climber, then a treadmill on an incline, and then a bike. You want to burn the most calories in the shortest amount of time. If you are really pressed for time, a quick run outside would also work because you won't lose the time going somewhere to work out.

Chapter 28

"Nothing can stop the man with the right mental attitude from achieving his goal; nothing on earth can help the man with the wrong mental attitude." —Thomas Jefferson

HEART RATE VERSUS FAT LOSS

I F YOU SEE AN OLDER heart rate chart in your local gym, you will see that most will have a "fat burning" and a "cardio" range. The "fat burning" range was based upon studies that looked at the first few minutes of exercise at different intensity levels. It is now accepted that the total amount of calories expended is more important than the intensity for overall fat loss.

Fat loss occurs over a 24-hour period, not just when we exercise. At the end of the day, it is still "calories in versus calories out." Exercise helps you increase your negative caloric deficit and helps to speed up your metabolism.

> It is now accepted that the total amount of calories expended is more important than the intensity for overall fat loss.

When you are exercising for cardiovascular and muscle endurance results, you must push yourself. There is a difference between activity and exercise if you want significant results, but for fat loss, all your body really cares about is negative calories.

For example, here are two possible choices for a workout. The first choice is to exercise on an elliptical trainer for 30 minutes and burn 500 calories. The second choice is to exercise on a bike for 45 minutes and burn 500 calories.

In both cases, you still have the same number of negative calories at the end of the day. Your overall "fitness" workout is better with a higher intensity, but weight loss would be similar.

Think of it this way. If you are a new runner and you go out and try to run as fast as you can for as long as you can, you may only last three minutes and burn 25 calories. It is intuitive that if you walked/jogged for half an hour you may burn 250 calories. It's clear that in this instance, the slower runner has the superior workout if the goal is fat loss.

You also need to be aware of the extremes with regard to heart rate and exercise. The rule of thumb is to subtract your age from 220 to get your maximum heart rate. Once you have calculated this level, don't exceed 85% of this number while exercising. If you are close to this number, you are close to your maximum safe level of exertion. There are exceptions to this rule, but for the majority of the population, this is a safe level of exertion.

> For example:
> 35 years old
> Maximum Heart Rate: 220 – 35 = 185 beats per minute
> Maximum Safe Exercise Rate: 185 x .85 = 157 bpm

Here is an easier, and perhaps more accurate way to determine your safe level of activity:

> While exercising, reach a sustained level of speed or intensity that makes you just breathless enough that you would find it uncomfortable to carry on a sustained conversation with a person moving alongside you. That is about the maximum safe level for many persons, particularly if not highly conditioned, and it is just above the level that will give you optimal heart, lung and circulatory conditioning. Of course lower levels can also be highly beneficial, and higher levels will be beneficial for those in good health training for competitive sports.

If you are exercising at a lower intensity and your heart rate is very fast, do not be too concerned. As your cardiovascular fitness increases, your heart rate will lower. If you are on a fitness machine that keeps your heart at a constant rate during exercise, you will find that over time, you will be working out harder and harder at the same heart rate.

LISTENER QUESTIONS

Q My question is about working out in the morning on an empty stomach. I have heard conflicting information regarding this. Some "experts" say you can burn much more fat by working out first thing in the morning before eating. Other "experts" say this is a myth. What is the truth?

A You are not going to lose more weight by working out on an empty stomach. It will seem that your workout is much harder because you will be low on energy, but at the end of the day it will not make a difference. You might technically burn some more fat during the workout itself without eating, but actual weight loss occurs over a 24-hour period and has to do with the "calories in and calories out" equation.

Some people find that they don't feel well if they exercise right after eating breakfast, so it might make more sense for them to hold off eating breakfast. However, without eating, you will have less energy. Consequently, you may not end up working out very hard, or even cut short your workout. As well, there is a lot of anecdotal evidence that working out on an empty stomach causes people to eat more later in the day.

The bottom line is, it doesn't really matter for weight loss. If for example, you eat 250 calories less and exercise an extra 250 more per day, you should lose about one pound per week regardless of when you exercise.

There is one crucial exception when you should always eat before you work out. Resistance training takes considerable energy, and you will not see a benefit if you are in a weakened state and are unable to truly push yourself. That doesn't mean that you have to eat a large breakfast. All that you need to do is eat a small portion of carbohydrates. Good food choices would include a banana, orange, yogurt or oatmeal.

Chapter 29

"The exercise is the spark and the food is the fuel, without both you'll see no flames—no results." —*Bill Phillips*

TO TRAIN AT HOME OR AT A GYM

TO HAVE A STRONG AND healthy body, a person must exercise. For long term success, exercise must include not only cardiovascular activities, but also resistance training.

Convenience may seem to be the most important factor, but over time, that may not be enough to motivate someone to use that equipment.

Whether a person chooses to train at a gym or at home is an individual decision. There are many personal factors that one has to look into before making a decision. It does not matter if one environment is "better" than the other. It only matters which environment a person will exercise in on a regular basis.

A person has to look at their lifestyle, commitments, personality, goals, finances, preferences, likes and dislikes etc. before even starting to evaluate which is better for them.

One important factor is convenience. Many people love to use their treadmill at home while watching television. There is no travel time or waiting in line at a gym for an available treadmill. However, some people quickly become bored with their treadmill and rarely use it after the first month at home regardless of how convenient it is. Convenience may seem to be the most important factor, but over time, that may not be enough to motivate someone to use that equipment.

In both cases, there is also the financial cost. A gym membership will have a monthly commitment and quality home equipment can cost thousands of dollars. After a year or two, the financial costs will most likely be the same. If you continue to use your home equipment for years to come, you are far ahead financially. If you don't, you are much further behind.

Here are some practical suggestions to find out where you belong.

1. **Rent before you buy.** Before purchasing a piece of equipment for the home, rent one for several months. If after a few months, you find that you rarely use it, you can return it. Even if you don't rent exactly what you are looking to buy, you will still see if working out at home is for you.

2. **If you choose to buy equipment for the home, look for used first.** The majority of used fitness equipment is for sale because it was rarely used. That two-year-old treadmill may only have 20 miles of use on it, but it could be $1,000 less than a comparable new model.

Where you are most comfortable, motivated, and likely to exercise on a regular basis is the most important factor to consider.

3. **Do not only buy cardio equipment for the home.** It is also important that you have the ability to do resistance training as well. Simple things like a chin-up bar, adjustable dumbbells and a weight bench are a good start. Larger resistance machines like a Bowflex are also an option, but they are also quite inexpensive if you buy used.

4. **Try before you buy.** Look for trial memberships or a monthly pass to try out some local gyms. All gyms are not created equal or cater to the same types of people. At a minimum, you will be able to try out all of the current fitness equipment that you may want in your home gym later on.

Where you are most comfortable, motivated, and likely to exercise on a regular basis is the most important factor to consider. Don't feel pressured to never switch. In the future, many people will outgrow their home gyms after a few years and want more variety in their training. Moving to a larger fitness facility now makes sense. Other people may realize after a few years of training at a gym, that they now have the motivation and drive to continue their program at home.

LISTENER QUESTIONS

Q If I am still sore the second day after my workout, should I still work out with my scheduled fitness class or should I only do cardio until I am not sore anymore?

A This is a question that is hard to give definitive advice because it is a dangerous question. You might think that you are sore, but this pain could ultimately signify an injury. You have to be aware of your own body and if you think that it is something more than soreness, you need to stop exercising and let it heal.

The muscle soreness that you are talking about is called DOMS, delayed onset muscle soreness. It starts 12 – 24 hours after exercise and can last up to a week. This is not the same as an overuse injury or other acute muscle injury that happens suddenly.

DOMS occurs typically when you do something that you are not used to doing, and then suffer later. For example, if you help someone move a lot of heavy furniture, you will probably wake up with sore muscles the next morning. Another example is when a "couch potato" signs up and takes their first intense "bootcamp" class. They may end up being sore and tender all over their body for several days. This is classic delayed onset muscle soreness.

You just have to listen to your own body. Nobody wants to train in a continual state of soreness.

The best way to avoid this is to gradually get into a workout routine. If you decide to take up running and do a 10-mile run the first day, you probably will not be able to get out of bed the following day. After a year following a reasonable, progressive running program, most people will be able to build up to running that distance without too much discomfort.

To answer the specific question about whether you should work out if you are still sore the *second* day after a workout, it should be safe. There are studies that show you can cause further swelling and pain if you work out the next day, but by the second day you should be safe to start easing back into it. You just have to listen to your own body. Nobody wants to train in a continual state of soreness.

You should start by doing a good warm-up to that area and do some light stretches. You will probably find that the pain will go away once you are warm and start working those muscles. The good news is that your body will adapt quite quickly and this soreness will not be something that happens for very long.

But remember, if you are in pain during an activity and it started suddenly—that is an injury and you need to stop your activity.

Chapter 30

"Most people's lives are a direct reflection of the expectations of their peer group."
—*Anthony Robbins*

HOW TO CHOOSE A GYM OR FITNESS FACILITY

I F YOU ARE PLANNING ON purchasing a new car, most people will go to many car dealerships and "kick the tires" on many comparable cars. This should also be done when purchasing a gym or fitness facility membership. Gyms can offer a wide variety of amenities and services. The goal is to find a gym that you will feel comfortable in, meet all of your needs, and will help you achieve your health and fitness goals. We recommend that you tour at least three gyms before you make a decision.

There are five major types of gym organizations out there:

Major national chains like Bally's. Depending on the type of membership you purchase, you may have access to all the chain's locations or just the ones in your local area.

Regional chains, like Sports & Health and Crunch, can be a great value by having more than one location in your area.

Franchised gyms like Gold's Gym, World Gym and others are national brands, but are individually owned.

Community organizations and cities often create recreation centres and offer their facilities to local residents. Because they are often tax supported, they may be less expensive and may have amenities like pools, ice rinks, and indoor sports fields that are cost prohibitive for private facilities to own and operate.

> We recommend that you tour at least three gyms before you make a decision.

The last type of gym is the **independently owned and small group facility**. The smaller gyms may offer better services and more opportunities to work with a trainer one-on-one.

When you are comparing gyms, these are the four things that you should be evaluating. A good gym should be able to meet all of these needs.

1. Equipment and Amenities

Is there a wide variety of equipment for both resistance training and cardio? Do they have a wide range of both free weights and machines to be able to work all of your muscles in different ways? Do they have many types of cardio machines to keep you from getting bored and enough machines so that you won't be waiting in line to use them? Is the equipment old or is it new and high tech?

> If the people working out around you are all huge bodybuilders and you're just starting out, maybe it's the wrong place for you.

There are gyms out there where every single piece of cardio equipment has its own TV and entertainment system built into the console! Talk about taking away the boredom from the treadmill or stationary bike.

For some people, the personal services and classes are most important. Are there personal trainers and nutritionists available? Do they offer a wide variety of group fitness classes that you find appealing and are offered at convenient times? Do they offer massages, tanning, snacks, juice bar, etc.? For families, on-site babysitting and children's programs may be important.

2. Location and Hours

One of the biggest factors that will determine how often people use their gym is the location. The location must be convenient for your lifestyle. Many people think that the best location should be halfway between your work and home. That way, you can either get up early and exercise, or go immediately after work on your way home. The hours of operation vary between gyms and range from being open only a few hours each night to ones which are open 24 hours. You should be aware that most gyms get a "rush" the hour before they close.

3. Atmosphere

This may be the most overlooked aspect of picking a gym. If the people working out around you are all huge bodybuilders and you're just starting out, maybe it's the wrong place for you. If you're a woman, you may find that you are more comfortable in a women-only gym. Does the gym have blaring techno music with annoying teenagers swearing and yelling or does the atmosphere seem clean, friendly and professional?

One component of atmosphere is whether you have friends that frequent that gym.

Having a workout partner or simply some familiar faces to say hello to can make the gym experience more enjoyable.

4. Price

In general, you get what you pay for. The better the facilities and services, the more it will cost. When comparing the prices of gyms, you need to study the contracts carefully to do an accurate comparison. There will be differences in enrollment fees, monthly or weekly dues, and length of the commitment. In a private gym, most of these things are negotiable if you ask. Also, make certain that the salesperson is aware that you are comparing prices of gyms in your local area.

Keep your eye out for promotions. Gyms often have promotions such as half off activation or enrollment fees or the first three months half off, or one month free. There are also discounts for paying up front for a year of membership instead of having your checking account debited.

Our final recommendation when trying to choose a gym, is to try before you buy. Most gyms will offer you at least a few free passes to experience the gym. Make sure that you show up at a variety of times and experience all of the amenities that you can.

Chapter 31

"A man may fall many times but he won't be a failure until he says someone pushed him." —Elmer G. Letterman

CARDIO: THE BASICS

C ARDIOVASCULAR EXERCISE IS ANYTHING THAT elevates your heart and breathing rate for an extended period of time. Basically, cardio makes you sweat and is great for burning off body fat.

A general recommendation for healthy living is to do cardio at least three times per week for 30 minutes each session. The more you do, the more calories you will burn, and the more fat will melt away.

This does not necessarily mean that you must go to a gym and use a treadmill or exercise bike though. Healthy activities such as rollerblading, cycling, hiking, swimming, jogging or even a brisk walk are all cardiovascular exercises. Here are some of the benefits of doing regular cardio:

1. **Burning calories.** Any exercise that burns extra calories will help you lose fat.

2. **Increase your metabolism.** The faster your metabolism, the more calories you will continue to burn even when you are not exercising.

3. **Improve your mood.** Exercise is a recommended treatment for depression. It simply makes you feel better by doing something physical.

4. **Sleep better.** Who doesn't want to sleep better? Some people find it difficult to sleep right after exercising, so you may need to exercise a few hours before you go to bed.

5. **Disease prevention.** Exercise reduces the risk for several diseases including heart disease, adult-onset diabetes, high blood pressure or hypertension, breast cancer, osteoporosis and colon cancer.

How hard should you train for maximum cardiovascular benefit?

You should train between 60 and 85% of your maximum heart rate to get the most cardiovascular benefit out of cardio training. A 30-year-old's maximum heart rate is 190. The low-end heart rate would be 114 beats per minute ($190 \times 60\% = 114$). The high end would be 162 beats per minute ($190 \times 85\% = 162$).

You will notice that when you first start out, your heart rate will be very fast while exercising. The more fit you become, the slower your heart rate will be at the same intensity of activity. Your resting heart rate will also drop as your heart becomes stronger. The average resting heart rate for an adult is between 60–70 beats per minute. A top marathoner's resting heart rate would be in the 40–50 range.

How to check your heart rate

The simplest way is to use a watch or timer and feel your pulse on your wrist or your neck. You will get the most accurate result by counting beats for a full minute. You could also count for 15 seconds and multiply your result by four. The problem with this way of checking your pulse is that you need to stop exercising to measure it.

A common tool, especially used by runners to check their heart rate, is a heart rate monitor. These are available at most running stores, pharmacies, and some sporting goods stores. A strap is fastened around your chest to sense your heartbeat. You then wear a special watch that is linked wirelessly to the strap around your chest. To see your pulse at any time, you simply look at your watch.

The more fit you become, the slower your heart rate will be at the same intensity of activity.

The final way to check your heart rate is to use exercise equipment that has a heart rate monitor built into it. The most common place to see a heart rate monitor is where you would normally hold on to the machine. These usually look like a strip of metal incorporated into the handle. For example, while riding an exercise bike, if you hold onto the handlebars, the handlebars will have the sensor in them and they will measure your pulse through your palms.

How often and how long should you do cardio?

Depending on the intensity that you exercise, and your specific goals, you should spend 20 to 60 minutes per session. After 60 minutes of exercise, you will quickly start to lose the benefits of it as you tire.

For maximum fat loss, the recommendation would be four to six days per week. If you have the time and the dedication, some people will even do two cardio sessions in one day. It is important though to make sure that you have at least one rest day per week.

Keep in mind, you will always burn the most calories doing something that you like. Even if you are doing an exercise that burns an incredible amount of calories per hour, if you don't enjoy doing it, you will simply not end up doing it.

LISTENER QUESTIONS

Q I just began a running program and I'm experiencing painful side stitches about 15 minutes into my run. Do you have any advice on how I might be able to prevent these from happening?

Safety first: It might not be a classical "side stitch." See a doctor immediately if the pain you experience emanates from beneath the breastbone or in the neck or radiates down the left arm, and is accompanied by shortness of breath.

A Side stitches generally happen to people when they first start doing cardiovascular exercise, but most people seem to "outgrow" them with continued training.

A side stitch is believed to be a cramp in the diaphragm, the large, flat, muscular membrane that separates the chest and abdominal organs and helps force air into and out of the lungs during breathing. Exactly why the diaphragm spasms, however, remains unclear. It seems to happen more with running than with other activities. One theory has to do with the timing of your breathing with the pounding of your steps, another is the sloshing of your internal organs because you have too much fluid in your belly .... but there are many theories out there.

The ways to prevent side stitches include gradually increasing the intensity of your workouts, breathing deeply as you exercise (not short shallow breaths), and strengthening your stomach muscles.

If you are experiencing a side stitch, this is Jeff's best solution that he uses in his Phys. Ed. classes. Hold both of your hands high above your head and walk slowly while taking five deep breaths. The goal is to relax, and do a little bit of a stretch so that the diaphragm will stop cramping.

Chapter 32

"Try not. Do or do not. There is no try."
—*Yoda in The Empire Strikes Back*

THE BEST CARDIO EXERCISES FOR FAT LOSS

F YOUR GOAL IS TO burn calories at the gym, you must be aware that all cardio equipment is not created equal. If you want to have the most productive workout in the shortest time, you need to choose the right equipment.

Here are the basic forms of cardio machines that you will see in health clubs or that you may wish to purchase for yourself.

Running—Outside or On a Treadmill

If you are running or walking outside on fairly flat terrain, you will burn more calories the farther you go. A 150-pound person will burn about 110 calories per mile, and you will burn more or less depending on your bodyweight. Whether you are walking or running, it is the distance that is important, not the speed in relation to the amount of calories burned. Of course, you will be done your workout sooner if you run.

If you are using a commercial grade treadmill, you will be able to enter in your bodyweight to get an accurate reading of the amount of calories that you burn. If you adjust the incline level so that you are moving uphill, you will burn more calories.

An average person may burn up to 350 calories in half an hour while running (six mph or faster) on a flat surface. If you walk briskly (four mph) at a 15% incline, you can burn more calories than running. You don't have to be a good runner to get a great workout from a treadmill.

Exercise Bike

Historically, this has been the most popular piece of exercise equipment at the gym and at home. Everyone has ridden a bike in the past, and it is not unfamiliar or awkward feeling when you first start using it. Many people read magazines or books while they ride to help pass the time. Most people find that when they are cycling at a challenging pace, they will burn about 300 calories in half an hour.

Stair Climbers

These used to be the most popular piece of equipment 15 to 20 years ago. There is an advanced stair climber in some gyms called a Stepmill. The Stepmill is just like walking up a real set of stairs. It is a mini escalator that runs backwards and you have to keep walking up it. It burns an incredible amount of calories, but most people find it too challenging after a few minutes.

Even regular stair climbers burn more calories than a treadmill or an exercise bike and are easy on your knees. The key points to remember so that you maximize your workout are:

1. Make sure that you are taking big steps—not just two little ones!
2. Don't support your body weight with your hands—you lose most of the benefits.

Most people will average about 350-400 calories in half an hour.

Elliptical Trainers

These are by far the most popular cardio equipment in fitness facilities today. It does take a few times to get used to the motion of the machine, but it is well worth it. Because you are using your legs and arms at the same time, you are exercising more muscles at the same time, and you burn an incredible amount of calories.

The main reason why people like this machine is because it seems like an easy exercise. When you monitor your heart rate, it will be elevated, but it will not seem that you are working very hard.

Because you are using multiple muscles at the same time, the elliptical trainer seems easier, people work harder, burn more calories, and burn more fat in less time.

Because you are using multiple muscles at the same time, the elliptical trainer seems easier, people work harder, burn more calories, and burn more fat in less time. It is not uncommon for people to burn 450-500 calories in 30 minutes on an elliptical machine.

Aerobics, Step Classes, Spinning Classes, Tae Bo, Pilates, Yoga, or Other Group Exercise

For the person who enjoys working out in a group, there are a wide variety of choices that you will discover at fitness facilities. Depending on the level of the class, these workouts can be challenging for even the most fit. As well, many of these classes incorporate muscle building exercises and cardiovascular work.

You cannot look at a class the same way that you look at a workout on a piece of fitness equipment. There is more of a social and support aspect than there is when you work out on a stair climber. If you have a hard time getting yourself to the gym, regularly scheduled fitness classes may be the answer for you.

Conclusion

Regardless of the type of cardio that you choose to do, to be effective you must put in a significant and consistent effort.

Chapter 33

*"Our growing softness, our increasing lack of physical fitness,
is a menace to our security." —John F. Kennedy*

RESISTANCE TRAINING IN A NUTSHELL

R ESISTANCE TRAINING IS ONE OF the most neglected portions of many weight loss programs. It is true that cardiovascular exercise burns more calories while you are exercising, but resistance training burns more calories after. It also speeds up your metabolism, which allows you to burn more calories all day long, even while you sleep.

Many women believe that resistance training will make their muscles too large and they don't want to bulk up. In reality, lifting weights will help them lose the fat layer that covers their muscles, and will leave them toned and defined.

The worst thing that you can do while losing fat is lose muscle at the same time. Muscle burns a lot of calories every day, even if you are not exercising. If you lose muscle, your body will not burn as many calories as it used to, and it will be easier to gain the weight back later on. You can think of weight training as insurance against muscle loss.

You can think of weight training as insurance against muscle loss.

Most people do not train to look like bodybuilders. They want to look like either the male fitness models who are on the cover of *Men's Health* magazine or the female fitness models who are on the cover of *Shape* or *Oxygen*. All of these models, male and female, do resistance training to attain the bodies that they have. If you want to look like a fitness model, you must eat and train like a fitness model.

There are literally hundreds of books that you can read on weight lifting and bodybuilding. There are also hundreds of variations of workout routines and thousands of exercises that you can perform.

Here is a summary of resistance training principles:

1. You tear down muscle to build up muscle

When you resistance train, you cause microscopic tears in your muscles. As your muscles heal these microscopic tears, they adapt to the strain of weight training and get larger as they become stronger. It should not be painful to lift weights. You will feel the "burn" of lactic acid building up near the end of a set, but you should never feel acute pain. Acute pain is a sign of an injury.

When you first start out, it is very common to experience muscle soreness that starts the day after (or even the second day after) and can last up to a week. This is known as delayed onset muscle soreness or DOMS. Working out too hard at the start causes this. Your body needs some time to get used to this type of training. It is better to train lightly at the start, than to overdo it.

2. You need to use challenging resistance

A rule of thumb is to choose a weight that is at least 60% of your maximum. You need at least this amount of weight to challenge your muscles to grow. If you can lift a 100-pound weight, you need to choose a weight that is at least 60 pounds.

For general resistance training, you should be able to lift a weight at least six times. If you can't, lower the amount of weight.

3. Sets and repetitions

If you lift very heavy weights only a few times (one to four reps), you will be training mainly for strength. Olympic weight lifters train this way. You will gain in strength, but you will not get large increases in muscle size.

If you train with light weights and do many repetitions (20+), you will be working on muscle endurance. This does not tend to burn a lot of calories or have much of an impact on the muscle. Lifting a five-pound weight 100 times will not have the same impact on your muscles as lifting a 25-pound weight eight times.

The standard for most programs is around three sets of six to 12 repetitions. Weight lifting fads come and go, but most people tend to come back to the basics. If you can't lift a weight at least six times, you should lower the resistance. If you find that you can lift a weight easily 12 times, it is time to increase the resistance.

4. Keep your sessions short

The maximum time that you should spend resistance training is 45-60 minutes. After an hour, you will be too tired to get any more benefit out of your workout. If you can't get in all of the exercises that you want to, split up your workout over two days.

If you are going to combine some cardio exercise such as stair climbing or treadmill, do this after you weight train. Doing cardio before will impact how much energy and strength you have.

5. Keep your rest intervals short

Do not rest more than 60-90 seconds between sets. This will keep your heart rate elevated and keep your workouts short. If you are bored between sets, do something proactive such as stretching or do a lap around the gym.

6. Every workout needs to be just a little harder

This concept is known as overload and progression. Your muscles will respond and adapt very quickly to whatever workout routine you throw at them. The amount of resistance that you lift today, may seem very light a year from now.

You don't have to increase the amount of weight that you lift every workout; you just need to increase the intensity. Other ways to increase the intensity would be to shorten the time that you rest between sets, or increase the number of sets and reps.

For example, you could start by lifting 25 pounds for three sets of six repetitions and rest 90 seconds between each set. You could gradually build up to lifting 25 pounds for three sets of 12 repetitions and rest 45 seconds between each set. Now you could increase to 30 pounds and start the process over again.

7. Do simple compound muscle exercises

When you have a choice between two exercises for the same body part, choose the exercise that you can lift the most weight. Most people choose the opposite and do the easier exercise that isolates a single muscle, but they do not get the optimal results. This way you will be training more muscles at the same time, and get the most benefits.

For example, using a seated leg extension machine works your quadriceps. However, if you do barbell squats, you will actually work most of the muscles in your legs and torso at the same time.

8. Your muscles grow when you are resting

This may not seem to make sense for many people, but someone who trains every day will get very poor results compared to the person who only lifts a couple times per week.

Remember that when you lift weights, you cause microscopic tears to the muscle. If you don't give the muscle time to recuperate, you will just keep tearing it and it never has a chance to repair and grow. When beginning, you can work the same muscles every day. As you become more advanced and use more resistance, your body will need more time to rest. Most advanced bodybuilders exercise the same body part no more than every six or seven days.

9. There is no perfect training program

Your body will eventually adapt to any program and your results will soon start to suffer. Don't get caught up in following a program that no longer gives you the results you want. If you change your workout once and a while, your body can't fully adapt to it and your results will continue.

The more experience that you have resistance training, the more quickly your body will start to adapt to any training program. But don't worry, if you really love a certain training program, you can always cycle back to it later.

Resistance Training Routines

Your body takes time to adjust to the demands of resistance training. It may take years of training for people to be able to handle an advanced program. Here is the basic progression that bodybuilding routines follow.

Level 1 Beginner

Most people start out by doing full body workouts. Most gyms will have a variety of machines that will train all of the major muscles of the body. Simply go to each of the machines and do one or two sets each. You can regularly train this way every second day.

Level 2 Beginner

Split your upper and lower body parts. This is known as a two-day split. One day only work your legs, and the next day work your upper body. Most people use mainly weight machines.

Level 3 Intermediate

Introduction of more free weights and perhaps new styles of routines. This is usually still a two-day split, but you may do more than one exercise per body part. One example of a routine would be a pyramid structure. This routine begins by lifting light resistance for many repetitions. As the routine progresses, heavier resistance is used with lower repetitions.

Level 4 Intermediate

A three-day split may be introduced. It now takes you three workouts to get through all of your body parts. You now do more exercises per body part, and you also get more days off before you work the same body part again. Many recreational body-builders stay at this level.

Level 5 Advanced

A four-day split is now common. Generally you will now have six or seven days off between the same body part. Workouts are very intense and you will need a week to recover. Most serious recreational bodybuilders stay at this level.

Level 6 Super Advanced

This is really for the professional bodybuilder who makes training their full time job. They may train as little as one body part per workout. They often train with weights two times a day, one body part in the morning, and one at night.

Conclusion

You don't have to do "trendy" routines to get a huge benefit out of resistance training. If you are new to resistance training, ask a trainer at a gym for a basic orientation. Just by following this simple advice, you should quickly start to see positive changes in your body.

LISTENER QUESTIONS

Q Is it possible to lose fat and gain muscle at the same time?

A To lose fat you must be in a calorie deficit and to gain muscle you need to be in a slight calorie surplus. That means that technically, you can't gain muscle and lose fat at the exact same moment.

But that does not mean that you shouldn't do resistance training while losing fat. Resistance training releases hormones that help you to hold on to muscle. The muscle mass throughout your body is what drives the speed of your metabolism, so don't lose muscle at any cost!

The least important thing while reducing fat is the speed of fat loss. The most important thing is that you don't damage your metabolism along the way

For the vast majority of people, there will be no true muscle gain while losing fat, especially if you are eating very little. However, the closer you are to your maintenance level, the higher the probability of gaining muscle while you lose body fat.

To improve the likelihood of gaining muscle, you must follow the principles that bodybuilders do. They eat every three or four hours, usually five or six meals per day, and they always eat a lean protein with every meal. If you keep your calories only slightly below your maintenance level and eat like this, chances are you can build some muscle while losing fat.

Q I have lost quite a bit of muscle through dieting. Now that my body fat is where I want it to be, how fast can I expect to be able to gain that muscle back?

A A crash diet that results in a 100-pound weight loss in six months, will severely damage your metabolism. The amount of muscle that will be lost in this type of diet may take years of consistent resistance training to repair.

We can't give numbers as to the exact speed of muscle growth that you can expect, but here are the factors that will influence it:

1. **The lower your calories are, the harder it is to gain muscle.** It is very hard for your body to be in a tissue growth (anabolic) and tissue reduction (catabolic) state at the same time. That is why it is difficult to gain muscle and lose fat at the same time. With only a moderate

calorie reduction it is possible, but with very low calories, it is almost impossible.

2. **The longer you have been training; the harder it is to gain muscle.** When you first start resistance training, you can expect to have accelerated results for the first several months. However, there is a point after many years of training where you can reach the upper limit of your genetic potential.

3. **The older you are, the harder it is to gain muscle.** A 40-year-old man will never be able to put on muscle like a 16-year-old can. A person needs a lot of testosterone to put on muscle, which leads to the next point. A woman only has a small percentage of testosterone compared to a man, and that makes it much harder for women to put on muscle. It can be done, but they have to work much harder and longer to get the same results.

4. **Gaining muscle is a difficult process.** It takes consistency, dedication, and a lot of sweat and effort. You need to push yourself well past your comfort zone for your body to respond.

5. **To gain muscle, working out in the gym is only 30-40% of what you need to do.** Most bodybuilders agree that your nutrition program is responsible for up to 70% of your results. One person can be working out just as hard as the next person, but one of them can easily be getting double or triple the results simply by eating a typical bodybuilder's diet of six meals per day and eating a lean protein with every meal. You truly are what you eat.

So what would be the range of pounds of muscle that the average person could put on in a year? Like we said, this isn't an easy answer. One thing is for certain, the claims that supplement manufacturers make in fitness and muscle magazines are an exaggeration of what is really possible for the average person. For example, a claim that anyone can put on 20 pounds of muscle in a month isn't possible, even for someone abusing anabolic steroids.

An average 30-year-old man, working out hard and eating properly for an entire year may be able to gain five to ten pounds of muscle in that year. The average woman would be lucky to gain half of that. Someone eating below the Basal Metabolic Rate can lose this much muscle in a month or two.

Q   What are the benefits of slow speed strength training? Do you recommend
     that people do it?

A   There is no one perfect form of strength training. No matter what type of
     training you do, your body will eventually adapt. The real trick is to constantly
     change your resistance training routines to keep your body from adapting.

You can change many things around such as the number of reps, number of sets,
the amount of weight or resistance, or how much you rest between sets. What
most people don't consider is the speed of the exercise.

Slow speed strength training is a great form of exercise. Many people find it to
be their preferred type of resistance training, but all people can benefit from
"slow lifting" as part of their overall resistance training programs.

The most common mistake that people make while doing resistance training is to
perform the movement too quickly. Usually they are trying to lift something that is
too heavy, and they try to use extra body swing and momentum to help "cheat"
with the weight. This is often counter productive and dangerous. The vast majority
of all resistance-training injuries are cause by doing exercises too quickly and
without proper technique and form. The slower that you lift, the better your form
has to be, and the more muscle isolating each exercise will be.

How slow is this form of resistance training? You generally lift the weight for
two seconds, pause for one second and then slowly lower the weight for four
seconds. It is a very safe method of resistance training mainly because the
dangers of momentum are removed. For this reason, many trainers start people
on this form of training, especially older people. There have been a handful
of studies published on the benefits, and they have all shown that participants
gained strength without the risk of injury. It isn't for everyone, because some
people might find it tedious, but it is beneficial for everyone who tries it.

Q   What is the best way to tone your muscles?

A   The unfortunate thing about toning your muscles is that there is no such
     thing. The term muscle toning is simply an invention of the fitness industry
and magazines. Sure, you will hear trainers throw out that term, but they are just
telling people what they are expecting to hear. People have heard the term out
in the general public and want their trainer to do that for them. If you look at
a university level exercise physiology textbook, you will find muscle growth and

muscle atrophy, but nothing about muscle toning as a response to exercise.

In reality, people don't care if they are really "toning," they just want the look of what that is. The look of a toned muscle is a combination of three things. The most important thing is a reduction of body fat around the muscle so that you can see it better. You can't spot reduce body fat; this will just be a result of overall body fat loss.

The second thing is an increase in muscle size. Your arm will seem to be smaller, but there will be an increase in the amount of muscle with less fat surrounding the muscle.

The third factor is often referred to as muscle tension. As muscle is regularly being worked hard, it stays a little tenser and isn't totally relaxed. That for example, might give some people a little more definition in their abs and show off that six-pack a little more even when they aren't flexing those stomach muscles—or at least pretending not to flex.

To get that look of toned muscles, there are three things that you must do.

1. **Do a regular, progressive resistance training program.** You must be committed to this in order to maintain and build a little more muscle. Make certain that your program is challenging, but also make sure that you take regular rest days from the weights.

2. **Do regular cardiovascular exercise.** This is important to burn extra calories to get rid of extra fat that will make your muscles look soft. As well, being in better cardiovascular shape also improves your overall health and makes you look and feel better.

3. **You must eat a balanced, nutritionally dense diet.** Make certain that you eat lean protein with every meal, eat often throughout the day, and that you eat only moderately below your maintenance calories. Your nutrition is extremely important if you are trying to lose fat and improve the look of your muscles at the same time.

Chapter 34

*"You have to stay in shape. My grandmother, she started walking
five miles a day when she was 60. She's 97 today and we don't know
where the hell she is." —Ellen Degeneres*

WALKING FOR WEIGHT LOSS

W HY WALK? YOU HAVE TO start somewhere. If you have been sedentary for a long time, possibly years, then walking is a great place to start your fitness routine. There are a couple of good reasons for this.

Walking is free. There is no special equipment required. You walk right now, albeit just to and from the couch, but you know how to do it.

It's easy to start. You can walk out your front door and start right now and burn some calories.

Walking is one of those "gateway exercises" because it usually leads to other forms of exercise.

If your muscles, joints, and ligaments are not accustomed to sustained activity, this is the best way to toughen them up for more rigorous demands in the future.

> You don't have to run to get calorie-burning benefits.

Walking is exercise. You don't have to run to get calorie-burning benefits. If you walk for an hour, you will burn the same number of calories that you would if you ran the same distance. You will not burn the same rate of calories per minute during your workout, but at the end, your calorie burn will be the same. It is true that you won't get the same cardiovascular workout and you won't get the same afterburn effect, but you will burn calories that will help you lose fat.

No special shoes or equipment is required to get started. You can buy more comfortable walking shoes, but they are not necessary. You will most likely not be sweating, so as long as you have comfortable clothing you will be set.

Depending on the time of day that you walk, there are a few safety concerns that you should be aware of. If you are walking at night, be sure to wear some type of reflective clothing or put some reflective tape on your shoes and clothing. You want every driver on the road to be able to see you while you're walking. Also, the sun can do a number on your skin. As a general rule, when you spend long periods of time in the sun, be sure to wear a good sun block and hat to protect your skin.

There are several gadgets and extra gear that can enhance your walking experience. The first is an iPod or other type of portable mp3 player. You will have the choice of listening to music, podcasts or even audio books.

The second piece of gear is a pedometer. A pedometer counts your steps and with the extra information of what your stride length is, you will know how far you've travelled. There are very sophisticated pedometers that will give you extremely accurate distances based on GPS satellites, and some even include a heart rate monitor.

Many people have heard of running programs or classes, but there are also many walking classes and programs that you can sign up for. Walking classes are typically offered at running stores that offer running programs. The concepts that they cover are very similar to the running classes. They have an education portion each class and also a progressive walking program that builds on intensity and duration. Walking programs and classes lend themselves to being quite social and enjoyable for most participants.

Walking is a "gateway exercise" to other and more intense activities, but don't pressure yourself or let others pressure you into running or other more strenuous activities until you are ready.

Lastly, if you are severely overweight or morbidly obese, you may find that the walking programs are too much for you. Maybe the five-minute warm-up is all you can do. That's fine. You'll progress at your own pace but the key is to not give up.

LISTENER QUESTIONS

Q Does walking or running burn more calories?

A A common misconception is that you burn more calories when you go for a run compared to going for a walk—but this is not the case.

It is true that you will burn calories at a **faster rate per minute** if you run, but whether you cover a three-mile distance in an hour or half an hour, when you get to the finish line your body did the same amount of work.

The scientific way to look at Work is the formula: **Work = Force x Distance.** It takes energy to move your body over a distance. If your body burns 10 calories to move a certain distance, going five times farther will burn five times the calories regardless of your speed.

The biggest factor in how many calories you burn is your weight. The heavier you are, the more energy it takes to move your body.

The technical formula to figure this out is: **Kilograms x Kilometers x 1.036**
Here is the Imperial version: **0.76 Calories x Pounds x Miles**
Here is the Combination version: **0.47 Calories x Pounds x Kilometers**

> For example, here is the Imperial formula for a 150-pound person who walks/runs 3.1 miles:
> *Total Calories = 0.76 x 150 x 3 = 353 calories burned*

> Here is the combination formula for a 150-pound person who walks/runs 5 kilometers:
> *Total Calories = 0.47 x 150 x 5 = 353 calories burned*

There are benefits of moving your body at a faster rate. You will not get a cardiovascular workout by moving slowly, and you will not get any afterburn effect from a casual stroll, but if your concern is getting in some activity that will burn extra calories, walking works!

So if you are watching TV at home and using a treadmill, you can easily walk 5K or three miles in an hour without dripping in sweat, and still burn the same calories as a run.

Chapter 35

*"A journey of a thousand miles starts with the first step and
a journey of 100 pounds starts with the first ounce."* —Unknown

RUNNING FOR WEIGHT LOSS

R UNNING IS ONE OF THE most popular forms of exercise. Any time of the day you will see people out running. With little gear, running can be a part of your fat loss regimen.

No matter where you are in your fat loss journey, there are some basic pieces of equipment that you need. Shoes are the most essential piece of gear and where you should start. We suggest going to a "running store" to get evaluated and fit properly for a pair of running shoes. Employees at a general sports store may not be well versed or trained in fitting you properly.

Running is a sport and to properly participate in a sport, you should have instruction.

The next most important piece of running gear is socks. Standard white cotton socks are not appropriate for running because of the friction produced within the shoe. With a cotton sock, that friction will be directly transferred to your foot. Cotton socks also hold moisture and keep that moisture directly on your foot. Friction plus moisture plus foot equals blisters.

Purchase socks that wick away moisture from the foot as well as provide a friction free environment. There are multiple brands of socks on the market that meet this requirement. They are often made of man made materials such as polyester, and have two layers that reduce or eliminate the friction.

Clothes also need to wick away moisture from perspiration. This reduces the friction on the other parts of your body. All running stores and most sports stores will have clothing to fill this requirement. One brand name to look for is Coolmax clothing. One of the most common areas of friction on a man are his nipples. Heavy, wet cotton t-shirts are known to rub the skin right off the nipples.

Most people think that proper running technique is natural, but it really isn't. Running is a sport and to properly participate in a sport, you should have instruction.

Most running stores also offer running classes. In those classes, people learn how to run, how to train, and most importantly, how to avoid running injuries. Most courses will also have a goal at the end. One of the most common programs is a "Couch to 5K" class. At the end of the course, the participants will race in a local 5K event. If you look on the Internet, there are thousands of sites and forums dedicated to running. Particularly if you are a beginner, be sure to check out those "Couch to 5K" programs and podcasts. These programs take you from a complete novice to running 5K in as little as eight weeks. There are less ambitious programs such as the "Four Weeks to a Mile" as well as more ambitious ones that will help you train for a 10K, half or full marathon.

A great way to stay motivated for running is to sign up for an upcoming race. If you are following one of these programs, sign up for a 5K that happens to coincide with the end of your program. Register for the race early and commit your money as well as your body. Putting up that $35 for the entry fee could be the difference in whether or not you succeed. It may be only a small amount of money, but it's completely wasted if you don't compete.

When you are confident in your running proficiency, it might be time to join a running club. Running clubs are communities of other runners. They meet on any day of the week, and can pair you with a runner of similar ability. That pairing can help you progress and you and your partner can push each other to succeed. Be truthful about your abilities; it will become blatantly obvious if you overestimate your running abilities on that first run.

Most of all, enjoy running. It's something that you can do for years to come.

LISTENER QUESTIONS

Q Do runners burn more calories when they run outside on a cold winter day?

A People who live in warm climates can never appreciate how much effort it takes, and the dedication needed, to go outside and run on a cold winter day. You just can't put on a pair of shorts and a t-shirt and go.

This is the gear that Jeff will wear when running in temperatures below -4°F (-20°C): two pairs of socks (one wool, one wickable), windproof underwear, a pair of insulated running tights underneath a pair of sweatpants, two long sleeve t-shirts made of wickable material, a heavy fleece, a windproof outer shell jacket, a balaclava like hat that fully covers his face, a pair of thin gloves with a pair of mitts overtop of them, and a pair of running shoes with small screws screwed into the tread for grip on ice.

Running in the cold winter is a lot of extra work just to get ready to go running— so right there you have burned extra calories getting ready, and then when you come back, you have three times the wet clothing to hang up. If you are running in snow, you can end up expending many more calories similar to if you were running in deep sand.

The actual research says that cold weather itself does not increase calorie needs. You don't burn extra calories unless your body temperature drops and you start to shiver. When you are running, the weather can actually be tropical inside your exercise outfit regardless of how cold it is outside.

However, your body does use a considerable amount of energy to warm and humidify the air you breathe when you exercise in the cold. According to research, if you were to burn 600 calories while cross-country running for an hour in 0°F (-18°C) weather, you may use about 23% of those calories to warm the inspired air. In summer, you would have dissipated this heat via sweat. In winter, you sweat less.

The Army allows 10% more calories for the heavily clad troops who exercise in the cold.

The weight of your extra clothing can also burn extra calories. The Army allows 10% more calories for the heavily clad troops who exercise in the cold. You won't be wearing that much extra weight in clothing, but it will count for a few more calories burned.

So the good news is that if you run in the cold, you will burn more calories. Depending on just how cold it is, if you do a three-mile or 5K run that burns around 300 calories, the cold could add 20%, which would give you an extra 60-calorie burn. You do get rewarded after all for suffering in the cold.

Q I have recently started using a treadmill as part of my workout. I was wondering which burns more calories: a faster pace, but lower incline, or a slower pace and steeper incline.

A This is something that you can test and figure out for yourself. There will be a point where running and walking on an incline will burn the exact same number of calories.

The factor that makes the biggest difference is how much you weigh right now. The more you weigh, the more energy it takes to move and the more calories you will burn.

The most effective way to increase your calorie burn, whether you are walking or running, is by increasing the incline percentage. At a zero percent incline, or perfectly flat, it is almost like balancing yourself as the tread moves under you. As a general rule of thumb, an incline of 1% is considered equivalent to running or walking outside in the real world.

Here are the results of a test that Jeff did for himself. He tested how fast he was burning calories at different speeds and inclines. He kept track of the treadmill's calorie count over a minute.

For Jeff, walking at 3.7 mph at 15% incline is the same as 8.6 mph at 1% incline for burning calories. He can alternate between walking and running in this example and continue to burn calories at the same rate. By doing that, he is doing two workouts at the same time; one for cardio and one for leg endurance and power.

To say which burns more calories, depends upon which workout you can sustain for any length of time. One is not necessarily better than the other. In this example, they are both burning the same amount of calories per minute, but if you have weaker leg muscles, you may not be able to keep up with a steep incline. As well, if you don't have a high level of cardiovascular fitness, you may not be able to run as fast for very long.

The big misconception with treadmills is that you have to run on them. That is simply not true. By varying your speed and incline, you get a much rounder workout and use a wider variety of muscles. Also, when you use more muscles, you won't be as sore after, or have the same risk of getting an over use injury. You are simply spreading out the impact on a wider range of muscles.

There is so much that you can do on a treadmill instead of just going for a certain distance at a certain pace. Most people will find their workout a little more interesting if they vary their speed and incline throughout a training session.

Chapter 36

"You are the way you are because that's the way you want to be. If you really wanted to be any different, you would be in the process of changing right now." —Fred Smith

CIRCUIT TRAINING

T IS IMPORTANT TO DO both resistance training and cardiovascular exercise, if your goal is fat loss or overall health and fitness. If you want an efficient workout, try combining the two together.

Circuit training is a type of interval training in which strength exercises are combined with endurance/aerobic exercises, combining the benefits of both a cardiovascular and strength training workout.

A typical circuit training set up will have a variety of different exercise stations, which alternate between a strength and a cardiovascular exercise. The workout consists of going through the entire circuit of exercises. At each station, the goal is usually to exercise for a duration of time, but other goals may apply such as a number of pushups completed or distance on a stationary bike. The participants continue until they have passed through all stations.

Here is an example of circuit training:

Station 1: Running
Station 2: Push ups
Station 3: Jumping Jacks
Station 4: Sit Ups
Station 5: Stair Climbing
Station 6: Squats

Most gyms will have an area set up for circuit training. Look for an area with a variety of resistance training equipment mixed in with a variety of cardio equipment. If there is no organized group of exercisers working through the circuit, a person can usually jump right in at any time. Some gyms make it easy for you to pace yourself in the circuit through the use of large timing clocks or even colored lighting that will change on a regular basis.

One of the benefits of circuit training is that it can be done at home and with minimal or no equipment. There are many body weight exercises that can be done almost anywhere. Then alternate with any other activity that raises your heart rate. The outside world is also a wonderful place to create your own circuit training programs. A typical children's playground offers unlimited potential for exercises.

Here are some general guidelines if you are going to set up a circuit for yourself:

- You can train two to four times per week. As with resistance training, at least 48 hours should be left between sessions that work the same muscle groups.
- For general fitness, a resistance should be chosen that allows the station to be completed for the prescribed period of time (don't go too heavy or you won't last).
- Eight to 12 exercises per circuit is plenty.
- Each station should be between 30-90 seconds, with 30-90 seconds rest between each.
- Go through the entire circuit up to three times with a two- to three-minute rest between each complete circuit.

As your level of fitness increases, you can increase the intensity three ways:

- Increase the station time that you are doing the activity.
- Decrease the rest time between stations.
- Increase the effort of each activity—heavier weights, pedal faster etc.

Circuit training is a very effective workout to add into your exercise regime. A typical 30-minute workout will burn hundreds of calories and give you a great full-body workout.

One of the benefits of circuit training is that it can be done at home and with minimal or no equipment.

LISTENER QUESTIONS

Q What are some strategies to be able to run farther and faster, but not get injured?

A For the average person, if they train smart, they will be able to run a 10K or half marathon race without ever suffering a running injury.

There is also a phenomenon called the "runner's high" where even beginners can experience a feeling of being in the "perfect zone" while running.

The main reason why people suffer running injuries is because they either progress too quickly or simply overtrain. A person's cardiovascular endurance improves faster than their joint, ligament, tendon, and muscle durability. As you get better and stronger, it just feels good to be able to run farther and faster. For many people, they find that they also rediscover the outdoors and fresh air. Most runners don't overtrain because they want to work harder, they just get hooked on running. If you take a beginner's running class that is eight or 12 weeks long, after a month or two, the problem is not to get people to do their runs on their own during the rest of the week, it is keeping them from running too far.

There is also a phenomenon called the "runner's high" where even beginners can experience a feeling of being in the "perfect zone" while running. It is sometimes referred to as "moving zen" and long distance runners say this is similar to being in a meditative trance.

Here are some strategies to remain injury free:

1. **The best way to start a running program is to take a class or follow a structured program.** A very popular type of running program is called "Couch to 5K." If you search for this on the Internet, you will find several similar programs to follow. If you have never run before, follow the most conservative program that trains you over several months to reach the goal of 5K (3.1 miles).

2. **Rest is very important.** You cannot run every single day of the week. All running programs incorporate days of rest. If you want to work out, you can still do other activities other than running.

3. **The 10% rule.** Do not increase your weekly distance total by more than 10% in a week, and don't increase the distance of your longest run by more than 10% in one week.

4. **Vary your runs.** Don't do the exact same distance at the same speed over the same route over and over again. Do short and long runs at varying speeds and don't forget to run up and down hills. With more variety in your runs, you will use more leg muscles and spread out the work of the run over those muscles.

5. **Periodization** is important because you cannot increase the intensity of a workout forever. Generally four months is about the upper time limit. At the end of a four-month cycle, start the progression over again. The progression will start at a slightly higher level than the previous cycle, and the goal is that at the end of the new cycle, you will be at a new high point. Then you start it over yet again. This is key for people who run continuously all year. This progression is natural for people who run in several "fun runs" or races during the year. These runners will train for each race. They will peak at race time and then take it easy and gradually build up for the next one.

6. **Stretch after each run when your muscles are warm.** Any repetitive motion such as running will create tight muscles. Many runners are now using "foam rollers" to aid in massaging tight hip, leg and knee areas.

Chapter 37

Even if you are on the right track, you will get run over
if you just sit there. —Will Rogers

INTERVAL TRAINING FOR CARDIOVASCULAR ENDURANCE & FAT LOSS

F YOU ARE LOOKING FOR a workout that is very short but very productive, interval training is for you. Interval training is the fastest and best form of training to drastically improve your cardiovascular fitness and it also burns fat.

Even though it is a short workout, there are two main ways that it will help you burn fat. First, it is an intense workout so your body will continue to burn calories at a faster rate after the workout is over. Second, if you do the same workout day in and day out, your body will quickly adapt and start burning fewer calories during those workouts. When you periodically do interval training, it keeps your body from adapting to any one workout.

Interval training can refer to any cardiovascular workout (stationary biking, running, stair climbing, rowing etc.) that involves brief bouts at near maximum exertion interspersed with periods of lower intensity activity. It works both your aerobic and anaerobic systems during the workout.

This is intense exercise that will definitely put a strain on your body during short bouts of maximum effort.

It is recommended that you consult your doctor before you attempt to do any form of interval training. This is intense exercise that will definitely put a strain on your body during short bouts of maximum effort. Also, if you are fairly new to exercising, don't start with intense exercise. Get a base fitness level first, and then gradually introduce this.

Here is an example of an interval-training workout. We are going to assume that you are running, but it could be any cardiovascular exercise. This will be a 20-minute workout, but you will also need to do a warm-up before you begin.

Minute 1: 50% effort—Moderate walking.

Minute 2: 60% effort—Light jogging.

Minute 3: 70% effort—Starting to get hard to hold a conversation.

Minute 4: 80% effort—You can only talk in short gasps.

Minute 5: 90-100% effort—This is the ultimate level where you are sure that you can only do this for 30-40 seconds, and the last 20 seconds you will need all of your willpower to complete it. Your muscles will ache, your lungs will hurt, you can't seem to get enough oxygen, and you will believe that you are about to die. This is the definition of 100% effort.

Starting Minute 6, you go back to 50% effort and go through that cycle three more times.

The benefits of this form of training are the short duration, the high calorie burn, the afterburn effect which fires up your metabolism for a few hours after the workout, and it will drastically improve your cardiovascular fitness in a short amount of time. However, there is a higher chance of injury if you do not properly warm-up before starting, and it is common for a person's cardiovascular endurance to outpace their muscular endurance. In other words, you won't be winded yet, but your muscles may be exhausted.

This isn't something that you would do every day, but it does have a place in everyone's fitness program.

LISTENER QUESTIONS

Q Is it true that interval training burns fat for 24 hours after the workout has been completed?

A The concept of afterburn refers to an increase in the speed of your metabolism after completing a workout. It is a true effect, but the scale of it is often over exaggerated. It is one of these things that has been spouted from trainers for years, but when the scientific literature started to show that the effect was smaller than thought, it seemed to be ignored.

Your metabolism is fired up after a workout, but the over-

The concept of afterburn refers to an increase in the speed of your metabolism after completing a workout.

all effect will most likely be under 100 calories, but it is definitely better than nothing!

Here is a little secret. By doing interval training every once in a while, it will help all of your regular workouts. As your body gets used to your regular workouts, those workouts will get easier for your body, and you will start to burn fewer calories to complete the same workouts. By including interval training workouts, your body can't adapt to your regular workouts, so those workouts will continue to burn more calories.

There is one activity that is shown to have the greatest afterburn effect. Resistance training with heavy resistance. This will give you the greatest afterburn effect and for the longest duration.

Chapter 38

"I would rather attempt something great and fail than attempt to do nothing and succeed." —*Robert Schuller*

CROSSFIT TRAINING

C ROSSFIT IS A PROGRAM OF interval training where you do incredibly hard, intense workouts. The crossfit website was launched in 2001 and they boast over 650 Crossfit gyms. The gyms are not like a typical gym. They don't have fancy weight machines that isolate specific muscles. They are all about Olympic barbells, kettle bells, medicine balls and chin-up bars.

A Crossfit workout could range from 15-45 minutes per session—very quick but very exhausting. Workouts most likely consist of three different exercises that you do in a circuit. You may complete exercises to see how many repetitions you can do, or just to see how fast you can do the workout.

Crossfit is a training regime for overall strength, agility and all-around fitness. They boast that the Crossfit program is the principal strength and conditioning program for many police academies and tactical operations teams, military special operations units, champion martial artists, and hundreds of other elite and professional athletes worldwide.

> Crossfit is a training regime for overall strength, agility and all-around fitness.

There seems to be hundreds of different Crossfit workouts and the workouts change on a daily basis. One main training goal of Crossfit is known as muscle confusion. Your body is never allowed to adapt, so you get the most benefit out of every workout. A social part of Crossfit, is that everyone does the same workouts and publishes their results for everyone to see. There is a main website at www.crossfit.com that will tell you what the day's workout is. You can do it on your own, or at a Crossfit gym, and then post your workout results there.

Many crossfit gyms have their own websites where participants post their results and comments about the workouts. You will eventually do some of the workouts again and you will be able to look back to see how you did earlier, so you can chart your progress.

Crossfit is, quite simply, a sport—the "sport of fitness." There are actually Crossfit games where people compete doing these workouts. If you go to the Crossfit.com website and take a look at the videos, you will see people who are in top shape. They are not just thin, but also have the other parts of fitness that people don't really think about such as cardiovascular/respiratory endurance, stamina, strength, flexibility, power, coordination, agility, balance, etc.

So the big question is, does this work for weight loss and can the average person do it?

Crossfit is excellent for someone who already has a basic level of fitness and is looking at losing that last 20 pounds of fat and putting on some muscle.

Crossfit is excellent for someone who already has a basic level of fitness and is looking at losing that last 20 pounds of fat and putting on some muscle. It is also great for people who are motivated by being in a group. The camaraderie of a good group can push people to do some incredible things in their workouts. If a person has a very competitive attitude naturally, they will excel here.

Crossfit is not well suited for people who are very overweight or have a very low level of fitness. A basic level of fitness is needed before moving to these more advanced and demanding workouts. Workouts are done at 100% intensity effort, and the risk of injury for untrained muscles unaccustomed to these demands is very high. This is where you would go after you have a basic level of fitness and want to take it to the next level.

LISTENER QUESTIONS

Q In the past, I was very active in a variety of sports. I have taken a number of years off, and now I want to get back into those sports again. I have lost most of my fitness level and I realize that I'm not ready to start playing sports again. What is the best way catch up and get back in shape as quickly as possible?

A The fastest way to get back into shape is to train smart. If your body isn't accustomed to intense physical demands, don't jump right back in to where you were when you were in better shape. This is the biggest mistake that most people do, and they end up becoming injured and this sets them even farther back. Give your body a little time to adjust and then increase the intensity of your training gradually.

Here are some specifics:

1. Work out a progression of intensity starting at 60% of what you can now do, and gradually increase the intensity over several weeks. It should be very easy at the start. You are not only training your cardiovascular system, you also need to get your muscles accustomed to the training. Your cardiovascular fitness will return much faster and will easily catch up once the rest of the body is prepared.

2. You don't want to injure yourself or over train. It seems counter-intuitive, but doing too much too soon will not get you there any faster. Part of training is also resting. Your body needs time to heal and repair from all of the new demands on it. Many people find that are stiff and lose flexibility when they start training again. Don't forget to stretch after each workout. This will improve your flexibility, and also help your muscles recover from the training.

3. Once your muscles are accustomed to more physical demands, you are now ready to work on your cardiovascular fitness. The absolute fastest way to improve cardio is with interval training. Do a variety of interval training workouts to reduce the risk of injury, and to improve the range of muscles being worked.

4. Don't forget to train specifically for the sports that you want to play. Does your sport require you to have a strong core like judo or other martial arts? Do you need a lot of endurance for sports where there is a lot of running like many field sports? Do you need explosive power for only short durations? Look to see what physical characteristics are needed to excel in your sport and then look for ways to simulate those demands in your workouts.

Chapter 39

"Realize that there is no such thing as failure. Keep this in mind and you will achieve all that you conceive in your mind. You never fail, you simply produce results." —Wayne Dyer

DEALING WITH TRAINING INJURIES

ANYTIME THAT YOU DO PHYSICAL activity there is always some risk of injury. If you are new to an activity, there is a higher chance of injury. The 3 main types of injuries that occur during physical training are overuse injuries, over exertion injuries, and of course accidents.

Over Use Injuries are most common in endurance sports such as running, cycling and swimming. These injuries are simply caused by doing too much too soon. Generally, you don't want to increase your training by more than 10% per week. Your body simply cannot adapt quickly enough for the increased demands. Runners are very prone to a variety of over use injuries because a person's cardiovascular system improves much faster than their muscular endurance. After a month of running, many people feel that they can do a 10-mile run. Cardiovascularly, they may be able to complete this task, but most likely they will develop injuries in a variety of joints and muscles. These injuries are avoidable by including rest days and gradually increasing the intensity of workouts.

Over Exertion Injuries are muscle injuries that involve strains and pulls. It is similar to an over use injury in that something is attempted before the body is ready for it. One common mistake when doing resistance training is not doing a proper warm up of the entire body before lifting. Cold muscle is not as elastic and is prone to injury. A good warm-up would include at least five minutes of cardio followed by light resistance training on the muscles that you plan to exercise. A 100% exertion in running, swimming, weight lifting, etc should not be attempted until your body has at least a few weeks to adapt to the training. A bodybuilder can train to complete muscle failure and exhaustion every week without injury, but an untrained person who attempted this workout, would most likely suffer many injuries.

Accidents are generally caused by lack of attention. They could range from falling off a treadmill, running or cycling out in front of a car, twisting your ankle while jogging or dropping a weight on your foot.

How to Treat

Acute Injuries such as a sprain, pull or strain need to be dealt with immediately. The first thing you need to do is stop the activity. **RICE** is the standard recommendation for treatment and stands for **Rest, Ice, Compression**, and **Elevation.**

- Rest will prevent further injury and will allow healing.
- Ice will stop swelling. It constricts injured blood vessels and limits the bleeding in the injured area.
- Compression further limits swelling and supports the injured joint.
- Elevation uses gravity to reduce swelling in the injured area by reducing blood flow.

It is important to begin RICE as soon as possible after an injury. Use a sheet or towel to protect the skin and apply ice immediately. Next wrap an elastic bandage around the ice and injured area. Don't wrap this so tightly that you cut off the blood supply, but it should be snug. Leave ice on for about 15 minutes every three hours. Once the swelling decreases, you can begin gentle range of motion exercises for the affected joint.

Healing from Injuries

Healing from sports injuries can take some time. After swelling is reduced, healing is dependent upon blood supply. A good blood supply will help move nutrients, oxygen, and infection fighting cells to the damaged area to work on repair. Athletes tend to have a better blood supply, and heal faster than those with chronic illness, smokers, or those with sedentary lifestyles. Ultimately, healing time varies from person to person, and you cannot force it to happen.

Average Healing Times
   Sprained ankle—Minor: 5 days; Severe: 3 to 6 weeks.
   Mild contusion or bruising—5 days.
   Muscle pulls—A few days to several weeks. This is dependent upon the severity and location of the injury.

When to Return

Healing time for any injury can be longer if you return to activity too soon. You should never exercise the injured part if you have pain during rest. When the injured part no longer hurts at rest, start exercising it slowly with simple range of motion exercises. If you feel pain, stop and rest. Over time, you can return to activity at a very low intensity, and build up to your previous level. Increase intensity of exercise only when you can do so without pain. You may find that the injured part is now more susceptible to re-injury and you should pay close attention to any warning signs.

Prevention

1. Always warm up slowly before every activity.
2. Get proper instruction in proper body mechanics for resistance training.
3. Listen to your body. Pain is a warning sign and you should not work through pain.
4. Cross train in a variety of different activities.
5. Do not over train; make sure that you have regular days of rest.
6. Do basic stretching after the activity.

When to Seek Help

If you are concerned about an injury, seek medical attention. (A sprain and a broken bone can hurt the same amount.) If you experience any of the following symptoms, it is definitely time to see your doctor or specialist:

- Pain persists for more than two weeks in a joint or bone.
- You have "point tenderness." That is, you can cause pain by pressing on a specific area, but pain is not produced at the same point on the other side of the body.
- Any injury to a joint that produces significant swelling. If left untreated, joint injuries can become permanent.
- You cannot move the injured part.
- There is persistent numbness, tingling or weakness in the injured area.
- Your injury doesn't heal in three weeks.

Summary

We train for the cardiovascular health benefits, improving overall health, strengthening our bodies, lowering and maintaining body fat levels, and for cosmetic reasons. It is not a race to get there. Most of the problems are caused by too much, too soon or too hard, too fast. What is the rush? Are you planning on feeling healthy and fit for only the next year or two after you reach your goals or for a lifetime?

LISTENER QUESTIONS

Q What are some training tips for hot and humid weather?

A When training outside in the heat, there are some definite precautions that you should take. When exercising in warm weather, the blood vessels near the skin dilate to help the body cool. This forces the heart to work a little harder as it tries to get enough blood to the muscles. This causes your heart rate to elevate higher than normal.

The key is to minimize the risk of a heat related problems and still get the most out of that summer workout. Here are some tips to make exercise safe, but still effective during the summer months.

- **Stay hydrated**
  Before exercise: Drink eight ounces of water 30 minutes prior
  During exercise: Drink three to six ounces of water every 15 minutes
  After exercise: Drink eight ounces of water in the 30 minutes following
- **Back off intensity levels.** When training in the heat, you will not have to work as hard to elevate your heart rate. Use a heart rate monitor and adjust your pace accordingly.
- **Avoid training during the hottest times of the day.** Take advantage of the extra daylight. Early morning and evening hours can provide you with a window of cool weather to get in a workout.
- **Take your workout inside.** Exercising in an air-conditioned house or apartment can give you complete protection from the heat. An exercise bike, elliptical machine, treadmill, or a simple set of dumbbells can provide you with a great workout without going outside. Also remember that most gyms are fully air-conditioned.
- **Work out in the water.** Find a local pool and switch to swimming as your aerobic workout, or just do water aerobics in the backyard pool. Your local YMCA may offer classes to get you started. It's not just for senior citizens.
- **Keep your face and neck clear.** If you have long hair, pull it back and up. Remove all jewelry that can generate friction. Also remove any make up and allow the skin to breath.

> When training in the heat, you will not have to work as hard to elevate your heart rate.

- **Give yourself a couple of weeks.** The human body is an amazing machine that will adjust to almost any condition. Back off intensity levels as you allow the body 10 to 14 days to acclimate itself to the hot weather.
- **Train with other people.** Your workout buddies will notice if you are in trouble, even if you don't.

If you are working out in the heat and you're not feeling well, you may be experiencing hyperthermia, an elevated body temperature. There are three main types of hyperthermia related injuries:

- **Heat Cramps** Major symptom: cramps or tightness experienced in significant muscles such as calves and abdominals.
- **Heat Exhaustion** Major symptom: profuse sweating. Your skin will appear cool and clammy. Body temperature will still be at normal levels.
- **Heat Stroke** Major Symptom: dry red skin. Sweating will stop as your body tries to conserve water. Core body temperatures of 105°F (40.5°C) are possible, and can be life-threatening if left unchecked. Loss of consciousness is possible.

If you suspect that you are experiencing any of the above symptoms of hyperthermia, or nausea and dizziness, **stop exercising.** Get out of the heat as soon as possible and drink fluids.

Chapter 40

"Let us not be content to wait and see what will happen, but give us the determination to make the right things happen." —*Peter Marshall*

GEOCACHING

WORKING OUT DOES NOT ALWAYS have to be about getting in the gym and pumping iron. It also doesn't mean hopping on the treadmill and pounding out five miles. It can mean just getting out and being active. There are obvious benefits to those activities, but simply being active and having fun is also beneficial. One such activity that both Russ and Jeff enjoy is Geocaching.

Geocaching is a global game where individuals hide caches of "treasure." The location coordinates of the caches are then posted on a web site for others to find by using Global Positioning System (GPS) devices. It is like a game of global hide and seek. It doesn't cost anything to play, and all that you need is a device that is capable of using the GPS network. There are a wide range of devices that can do this, even some cell phones. It's grown in popularity and you should be able to find multiple geocaches within walking distance of your home. The health benefits come in when you strap on the hiking boots or walking shoes and head out to find a geocache. Not only will you be searching to find the cache, you will also be exercising at the same time.

Most caches will be hidden in public places like parks and recreational areas. Some geocaches are put into locations where you will have to hike a fair distance to find them. Others you can drive right up to and discover.

The health benefits come in when you strap on the hiking boots or walking shoes and head out to find a geocache.

To go geocaching, all you'll need is a handheld GPS device or phone with GPS capabilities and access to the website www.geocaching.com. Register for a free account, enter the coordinates into your GPS unit for your first hidden cache, and head out on your first treasure hunt. When you discover a regular geocache, it will be some sort of weatherproof container. Inside you will find a variety of prizes and a logbook.

When you discover a regular cache:

- Take something from the cache.
- Leave something in the cache.
- Write about it in the logbook.
- Hide the cache back where you found it.

Another type of cache is the location cache. When you go to the goal coordinates, you will find a picturesque spot to take a picture or have lunch with your fellow geocachers. Most of these amazing spots would never be discovered by people without the benefit of this sport.

A final type of geocache is a multi-cache. This a multi-stage treasure hunt. Each location that you find will provide the coordinates to the next location. Eventually, you will find the end of the trail and the final cache.

If you love the outdoors and are looking for something that encourages you to go out into nature and go hiking with a purpose, geocaching is something to look into.

MOTIVATION

THE THIRD PILLAR OF LIFE-LONG SUCCESSFUL FAT LOSS

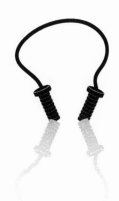

Knowledge is power, but in reality knowledge is only Potential Power. You actually have to get off your butt and do something to make anything happen." —*Jeff Ainslie*

STAYING MOTIVATED

YOU CAN KNOW EVERYTHING ABOUT nutrition and exercise, but you will not achieve a fit and healthy body unless you apply what you know day after day. Nothing was ever accomplished with only good intentions. Motivation is the key to sticking with your new fitness goals, but what can you do if you lose your motivation? Here are some truths about motivation:

Nobody besides yourself can motivate you. Ultimately, it is 100% up to you. You can hear a great motivational speaker that will fire you up, or find a great role model that you want to be just like, but that will only give a temporary boost in your motivation. When the daily grind starts to hit you, you will find that the only source of motivation that really counts is from within you.

The harder something is to do, the more motivation you will need. Losing 100 pounds in six months is exponentially harder than losing 100 pounds in 18 months. Anyone can be highly motivated for a few days, but most cannot do it for a few weeks or months at a time. Having said that, keeping your motivation level high for months at a time is also very hard to do. A person can learn techniques for improving motivation. By applying these skills, it is possible that you can make yourself more motivated.

We have five main points for anyone who is finds that they are falling off the wagon. These are definite things you can do to get fired up again.

1. Have powerful reasons that you want to lose fat.

Just wanting to be healthy or live longer are good reasons, but they don't give you an immediate urgency. You must seriously examine your life and situation and come up with some meaningful reasons. They also need to be reviewed on a regular basis to stay fresh in your mind.

Here is a practical suggestion of what you can do today. Write down a minimum of five reasons that all start like this: "I must lose body fat and become more physically fit, because if I don't.... (fill in the rest)." Come up with a list of reasons that are truly meaningful to you and can invoke an emotional response. The more powerful those reasons are to you, and the more often you review them, the better.

2. There is a simple mindset that you have to adopt: The pain of not losing weight should be more painful than going through all of the effort to get healthy.

Start thinking of all the negative emotions that being overweight brings up in you. Dwell on those emotions when you think of the temporary good feelings you will get from eating a donut. Then compare your few moments of enjoyment from the donut to all of those negative feelings that are with you every single day in your current condition.

The temporary good feeling from eating the donut cannot be as good as being fit and healthy. Nothing should ever be able to taste as good as being healthy and fit feels. People always do what they think is the easiest in the long run. If you start to realize that it is easier and more fulfilling to be healthier and fitter than feeling like a heavy, lazy slug, you will automatically have more fuel in your motivation tank.

3. Set many short term and daily goals.

Have a checklist of five to 10 things each day to accomplish. These are things that, if you do them, you cannot help but become fitter, healthier and thinner. Weight loss is all about doing these little things day after day that add up. Check those accomplishments off at the end of each day.

Let's say that you have 10 specific goals each day that you want to accomplish. If you don't make one or two, it isn't a failure. You can look back and still see that you made 80 or 90% for the day.

Just saying day after day that you are going to lose weight isn't enough. You must set easy measurable goals each day that you can do and succeed at. The bottom line is, you cannot improve what you cannot measure, and you can't feel great about accomplishing goals every single day, if you don't have daily goals to fulfill.

The next two points go together.

4. When you fall off the wagon, you just have to get right back on.

You must do it now. Never say that I will start again tomorrow—you must do it now. Momentum is the key.

Here is a common excuse that people use when they don't truly want to get back on track. They say "I'm going to start tomorrow, because I just blew it today and there is no sense starting until I can get a clean start." Or even worse, someone might say "Well, I'm not going to start my diet until I reach a nice even number of pounds. Why don't I wait until I reach exactly 200 pounds, because then it is easier to track how much weight I have lost"!

That type of thinking is all wrong; you need to start right now.

Even if you just had a horribly unhealthy lunch and say to yourself that "I already blew today, I might as well just blow the rest of the day and then start tomorrow"—it really doesn't matter. If you don't start now, you probably won't start tomorrow. That is the reality.

If you say that you need to go shopping for healthy food so that you can start tomorrow—that doesn't cut it either. When you are on track, you will still need to go shopping to get food—that is no excuse to eat like crap right now.

> **If you don't start now, you probably won't start tomorrow. That is the reality.**

The last point seems very simple, but it is the most powerful one. There are current studies that demonstrate that this is an extremely effective psychological technique.

5. If you can't seem to get back on the wagon, act as if you can, and go through the motions of being on the wagon.

You may have heard the expression "fake it, until you make it." The momentum will catch up to you when you start to see results again, and then you will not have to fake it, you will be back on track!

It is so simple and yet so powerful. Give it a try, there are no excuses. If you can't bring yourself, to act as if you are on the wagon, you need to act, as if, you can bring yourself to act as if you are acting as if you are truly on the wagon …We can go all day with this logic—just do it, suck it up, and it will work.

If it doesn't work, and you don't have your momentum back, what is the worst thing that will happen? You will weigh a few pounds lighter and be a little healthier. You have nothing to lose.

LISTENER QUESTIONS

Q Everyone seems to recommend that I should keep a food journal in order to lose weight. How important is it that I keep track of what I eat on a daily basis?

A Keeping a food journal is probably one of the most important things that you should do if you are trying to lose weight. If we could only give people one tip to improve their weight loss results, this would be it. According to research and published studies, dieters who kept food diaries lost twice as much weight as those who didn't. That is huge!

> According to research and published studies, dieters who kept food diaries lost twice as much weight as those who didn't.

Weight loss success or failure is not an accident. It is all about calories in versus calories out. While people think they know how many calories they are eating, most of the time they woefully underestimate.

On one episode of Fat 2 Fit Radio, we discussed a survey done at a Subway sandwich shop where patrons were asked to estimate how many calories they were eating. They estimated the number of calories at 350-400 while the real calorie count was closer to 1000. In our world of processed foods, there are more calories present in our foods than we think. By taking the time to create a food journal or by using online tracking tools, you will find out how many calories you are truly eating in a day.

Many people have managed to gain 10 pounds per year, by only eating 100 extra calories per day. In five years, they can easily gain 50 pounds by only eating an extra slice of bread each day. In a similar fashion, many dieters have failed to lose fat because they don't think that the calories in those little snacks and "tastes" of food actually count.

By keeping a food journal, there will be no mystery as to why you are successful or unsuccessful in your fat loss goals. If you truly track everything that you eat on a daily basis, it will make you accountable and conscious of what you are eating. Be honest and write down everything.

We always say that to have life-long success in weight loss, you simply need to live the lifestyle of that thinner person that you want to become. In many cases, the difference is only a few hundred calories per day. Keep a food journal for at least as long as it takes for you to learn what your goal number of calories looks like. This will make it easier and more effortless to mentally keep track of your approximate daily calorie intake into the future.

Chapter 42

"So what do we do? Anything—something. So long as we just don't sit there. If we screw it up, start over. Try something else. If we wait until we've satisfied all the uncertainties, it may be too late." —Lee Iacocca

ADVANCED WEIGHT LOSS TECHNIQUES

I F ARE LOOKING FOR A quick fix that will allow you to lose 10 pounds of fat this week, you will not find it here. We simply will not suggest things that might speed up weight loss for a few weeks, but will almost guarantee that you will gain all of that weight back. Our philosophy is long term. We simply don't care how much you will weigh in three days or three weeks. We care that you will reach your goal weight and then be able to report back year after year that you have maintained close to that goal weight.

Having said that, you can speed up your fat loss safely. These techniques generally take more effort—either physically or mentally and you will need to be more conscientious of what you are doing.

The bottom line is that you will always need to be working with the important caloric balance—calories in versus calories out, but you can certainly tweak things.

These accelerators work in conjunction with everything else that we suggest such as only doing a moderate calorie restriction, regular exercise, eating five or six times per day, eating mainly unprocessed foods etc. These techniques are also temporary accelerators that you can do for a month or two, but are not meant to be followed for the long term.

1. Zig-Zag

This technique is used when you want to increase your fat loss without the risk of slowing down your metabolism. What you do is lower your calories a little more than what we normally suggest, but then you add in a higher calorie day to keep your metabolism from slowing down.

Of course we are not recommending starvation levels, but let's say that you were eating at 400 calories below your current maintenance level to lose fat. You could increase the deficit by 50% to 600 calories. You would eat at this level for three or four days, but then the next day you would eat at your current maintenance level.

What you are trying to do is keep your body from noticing that you are losing fat at an accelerated pace. Your metabolism can slow down from eating too few calories or from long term dieting. By only eating at low calories for three or four days at a time before re-feeding your body, you can trick your body for a little bit longer.

Keep in mind this is only a temporary technique. The lower your calorie levels, the quicker your body will adapt to slow your metabolism. This may not help very much if you eat below your BMR, but it keeps your body oblivious to your fat loss for a little longer.

2. Double Cardio

To increase a caloric deficit, it is always better to increase exercise than it is to reduce calories. Double cardio refers to doing two sessions of exercise in a day, not just a longer workout. Doing two 45-minute sessions of exercise is more beneficial than doing a 90-minute workout.

Again, this is only a temporary thing, but it will boost your weight loss. This works for a couple of reasons:

- The longer a workout is, the less benefit you will get out of the extra time. This is known as the Law of Diminishing Returns. In a long workout, you get the most benefit out of the first half hour.
- After you work out, there is an afterburn effect, where your metabolism will stay elevated for a few hours and burn some extra calories. With two workouts, you will get double the afterburn effects.
- This reduces the risk of injury from overuse. Running four miles in one continuous run is not the same as doing two, two-mile runs with 10 hours of rest between them. The impact on your body is much less, but you will get the same caloric benefits.

This is definitely one thing that should only be done for the short term. It can surely help you lose a few extra pounds in the last month before a special event, but doing it for too long can lead to over-training.

3. Carbohydrate Cycling

This is similar to the zig-zag calorie technique, but you do this with carbohydrates. Low carbohydrate diets do have some positive advantages for weight loss, but they are not sustainable for most people in the long term. When people do not eat enough carbohydrates, most end up feeling very lethargic and don't have enough energy to work out effectively. After about three days on low carbs, the glycogen stores in your muscles will be depleted. If you then re-feed your body with good carbohydrates for a day, you will still have the energy needed to work out and feel energetic. The best part about these three techniques is that if you combine them together, you will get a nice acceleration in your weight loss. You are lowering your calories a little more with a trick to keep your body from noticing, you are increasing the amount of calories that you are burning by exercising more, and you are playing around with the percentage of carbohydrates that you eat.

LISTENER QUESTIONS

Q I weigh myself weekly and I try to eat the same calories every day, but some weeks I actually gain several pounds and others I have a huge weight loss. What is going on?

A This is an extremely common question. One week, we received an email from a man who tried out a new supplement and was extremely happy that his scale showed a 2.5 pound weight loss. He didn't change his eating habits and thought that the miracle supplement was responsible. The same week, we also received an email from a woman who estimated that she probably ate an extra 200 calories per day, but had gained 2.6 pounds in a week. They both wanted an explanation.

Weight fluctuations are natural and occur daily for most people.

The explanation is that everybody's weight will fluctuate for a variety of reasons, and you may not be able to pinpoint the reason for the fluctuation. Weight fluctuations are natural and occur daily for most people.

Some people are guaranteed to bump up three or four pounds on the scale if they eat salty movie popcorn—especially if they are not accustomed to eating a lot of salt. They did not gain three or four pounds of fat. They are simply retaining extra water weight because of the salt. When the salt is flushed out of their body, their weight will quickly drop again.

Even in the most controlled weight loss studies where people eat carefully measured amounts of food and exercise at a controlled intensity and duration, weight loss is never linear—there are always ups and downs along the way. Sometimes you will struggle to lose a single ounce for a week and then all of a sudden, your body seems to catch up. Sometimes you can seem to be working hard and your weight bumps up a bit. We are not machines, so you don't always get what you expect on a daily or even weekly basis.

It is natural for this to happen. What you need to do is keep track of your average weight over a week to remove these fluctuations. As long as your average is moving in the right direction, you don't have anything to worry about.

As long as your average is moving in the right direction, you don't have anything to worry about.

Remember, your goal really is not to weigh a certain amount, it is to be a smaller person. So make sure that you are tracking you measurements with a tape measure as well. If your weight fluctuates a couple of pounds, you will not see a difference in the size of your thighs or arms for example. If you are keeping track of your body fat percentage, you shouldn't see big fluctuations there either.

Chapter 43

"We can't solve problems by using the same kind of thinking we used when we created them." —*Einstein*

SUPPORT IN WEIGHT LOSS

O NE OF THE MOST IMPORTANT factors in the success of your healthy lifestyle is your support network. The people around you that encourage your efforts and make it their priority to help you are invaluable.

A support network is a group of individuals with a common goal that come together to talk, share information, vent, and otherwise encourage each other. Sometimes this encouragement can even take on the form of competition. On Fat 2 Fit Radio, the type of support network we usually discuss is the "diet" or "weight loss" group. These groups can take on many shapes. Locally it could look like:

- A Weight Watchers meeting
- Your local gym
- A community center
- Your church
- Neighbors or family members

The online communities are now incredibly popular. Instead of just your local area, the support groups span the entire world. A few popular places to find support online are:

- Yahoo! Groups
- Google Groups
- Bulletin boards
- Podcast communities
- Meetup.com
- Social Networks—Facebook, Spark People, Traineo, Live Strong

The online weight loss support industry is growing quickly in popularity. In November, 2007 a search on Google for "support in weight loss" yielded 29,800,000 search results. As of 2010, the same phrase received 51,300,000 search results.

While it's not impossible to lose weight on your own, a support network can make your fat loss more successful and enjoyable.

Start by taking small steps. We suggest to start by charting your weight or the foods you're eating on one of the online services mentioned. Then, when you feel more comfortable with the idea of sharing your information, explore online support forums like the one at fat2fitsupport.com. Read through posts and give some people a few words of encouragement. And finally when you're ready, ask a question that you have been dying to ask. As you gain more confidence and more knowledge, you can then help others new to the online group.

> While it's not impossible to lose weight on your own, a support network can make your fat loss more successful and enjoyable.

Remember that along with receiving support, you can also give support. A support group is a two-way street.

Here is one final suggestion of how to pull someone into part of your support group. This suggestion will also make you more accountable. Tell a friend the following: "If you see me gaining weight, ask me about it. I don't want to undo all the good that I've done for myself by losing this fat."

It is as simple as that. As you start losing weight and people notice, they will tell you. However, most people will not mention that they have noticed weight gain. Give that person, or multiple people, permission to call you on gaining back that fat!

LISTENER QUESTIONS

Q My question relates to cheat days. I have been attempting to eat more cleanly than I have in the past, but I simply can't give up some of the higher calorie and junk foods that I love such as pizza, hamburgers and movie popcorn. If I have a few "cheat meals" each week am I destroying my diet? Am I cheating myself out of sustained fat and weight loss, or actually encouraging productive metabolic boosting through such a practice?

A There are definitely two viewpoints on this. There is the textbook nutrition-ist/dietitian viewpoint, which states that if you eat perfectly with plenty of fruits and veggies and lean proteins and no processed foods etc, it is the most healthy way to live. If your goal is fat loss, eating this way will speed up your fat loss and be the most healthy way to do it.

The second viewpoint is less strict and is the one that we support. We don't encourage restrictive diets that will forever deny you of some of your favorite foods. The philosophy of "everything in moderation" is a strategy that people can follow for a lifetime. It really doesn't matter if you are on the best eating plan in the world, if you can't stick to it for more than a short time. For most people, following the perfect eating plan 90% of the time is much better in the long term and doable for a lifetime.

If your goal is losing fat and keeping it off for the rest of your life, then "cheating" can be beneficial.

Now to answer the question specifically. If your goal is to lose a specific amount of fat per week, cheating is counter productive to fat loss. If you add extra calories from cheat meals, it will affect the calories in/calories out balance.

However, if your goal is losing fat and keeping it off for the rest of your life, then "cheating" can be beneficial. If you want to keep the extra fat from returning, you need to live the lifestyle of that thinner person that you want to become. That thinner person still gets to enjoy the occasional summer barbecue, birthday party, wedding, or any other social event without guilt. That thinner lifestyle is one where the occasional indulgence doesn't hurt, because the other 90% of the time they are eating healthy.

We recommend eating five or six meals per day. Let's say that you eat five per day; that is 35 per week. Eating not-so-great foods for two meals per week still leaves you with 33 out of 35 good meals—that's 94% on task!

One last point, a cheat meal can be worked into a program and still hit your weight loss and fitness goals. Jeff regularly eats 100-150 calories less per day than his maintenance level during the week, so he can splurge a little bit on the weekends. Many programs allow you a cheat meal per week, but you don't want to go overboard and blow your entire week's calorie deficit. You can also make "better bad choices" and still enjoy some of the foods that are bad for you once and a while.

Chapter 44

"I have been impressed with the urgency of doing. Knowing is not enough; we must apply. Being willing is not enough; we must do." —Leonardo da Vinci

WEIGHT LOSS BLOGS

I F THE INTERNET DOES ONE thing well, it connects people. A fat loss journey doesn't have to be a lonely endeavor if you don't have a support group of people. The Internet can provide that support. For some time, people have been sharing their stories and life experiences in web logs, or blogs for short. A weight loss blog is one that shares the fat loss experience with others.

In general, a blog is a series of short articles, shown in reverse chronological order. The feature that makes a blog different from a series of articles, is the ability for readers to make comments on what they are reading. The experience is further enhanced with categories, tags, and keywords that makes your blog more searchable and discoverable by those looking to read what you have to say.

Why do you want to create a fat blog? In a word: **Accountability**.

When you create your own fat loss blog, you publicly announce to the world that you are entering a new healthy lifestyle. People around the world, who are interested in your experiences and ponderings about your fat loss journey, will follow your progress and comment on what you have to say. If you write it, they will come. But how do you create a blog?

There are now multiple easy ways to create a blog. Here are few of the numerous dedicated blogging services that will help you start your fat blog:

- Wordpress.com
- Blogger.com
- LiveJournal.com
- Tumblr.com
- Vox.com

Because fat loss blogging has become so popular among those looking to shed their excess pounds, there are now many sites dedicated to community and weight loss. These sites offer the ability to blog on their service as well. A main benefit is that you will already have a built in audience. Each person on these weight loss sites are there for the same reason that you are. What better place to start your fat blog?

Here are a some of the more popular services that offer blogging as just a part of their services:

- Sparkpeople.com
- Livestrong.com
- DailyBurn.com
- Traineo.com

If you don't want to write and publish your own experiences, help support others in their weight loss journeys. Being part of a community is motivating for all.

LISTENER QUESTIONS

Q How do you truly get rid of cellulite? Do any of the cellulite creams work or are there special forms of exercise that I can do to reduce my cellulite?

A Here is the truth; there is almost nothing that you can do to get rid of the look of cellulite. Men and women can both have cellulite. Cellulite technically is subcutaneous fat that pokes through the fibrous connective tissue that supports the skin. The reason why more women have cellulite is because their skin is thinner. Everyone has a level of fat beneath his or her skin and it is true that the more subcutaneous fat you have, the likelihood of getting cellulite is higher.

The only way to get rid of the look of cellulite would be to make the fibrous connective tissue that supports your skin thicker, and you can't do that. Having a large amount of fat isn't a guarantee that you will have cellulite and being thinner isn't a guarantee that you won't get cellulite either. Your genetics are the most important factor.

If you do have cellulite, losing fat will help with the appearance, but it most likely will never fully go away. The reality is, many people have cellulite. It is estimated that 40-50% of all female celebrities have cellulite. 100% of photos are manipulated to some extent before being published. That is standard practice in the media to do image manipulation, color correction etc. to every picture.

The unfortunate thing is that people believe that all of these celebrities look like this in real life, and try to live up to these unrealistic expectations. People have to realize that everyone has a genetic potential, and you can still be happy and content when you are the best that you can be.

Chapter 45

"The road to success is dotted with many tempting parking places."
—Author Unknown

TOPS (TAKE OFF POUNDS SENSIBLY)

M OST PEOPLE HAVE HEARD OF Weight Watchers or at least seen their commercial food products. But Weight Watchers comes at a hefty price. You pay to join and pay at each meeting you attend. Weight Watchers is a business. A business that will help you lose weight, but as with all businesses, the bottom line is not your waistline, it's their profit margin. There is an alternative though. It's a non-profit group called Take Off Pounds Sensibly, or TOPS.

From the TOPS literature: *TOPS Club, Inc. is a nonprofit, non-commercial weight-loss support organization based in Milwaukee, Wisconsin, USA, with chapters located worldwide. Its two-fold objective is to encourage healthy lifestyles through weight-management support groups and to sponsor obesity research.*

TOPS was founded in 1948, over 60 years ago, as a response to the need to assist overweight and obese people to lose weight by setting up a support group system. TOPS has about 170,000 members in nearly 10,000 chapters in the United States, Canada, and numerous other countries throughout the world. Membership includes men, women, and children. Dues are $26 annually in the United States, and $30 in Canada, plus nominal chapter fees to cover operating costs—on average, less than $5 per month.

With all businesses, the bottom line is not your waistline, it's their profit margin.

When joining, new members check with their doctor to obtain a goal weight for themselves. Members of TOPS meet weekly to do a private weigh in that is followed by a meeting. The weekly activities in a TOPS meeting will vary. Often members of the group will share a recipe or a story of their weight loss journey to encourage and inspire the other members. As well, many outside guest speakers speak at meetings. Contests, raffles and prizes are regular features of meetings.

To hold members accountable for their weight loss each week, they do a roll call activity. Each member will report their weight loss or gain for the week. Names of absent members are read off and the other members will "hold them accountable" for their weight at a later meeting or over the phone.

Meetings close with the following positive affirmation, or pledge:

> *I am an intelligent person. I will control my emotions and not let my emotions control me. Every time I attempt to use food to satisfy my frustrated desires, build up my injured ego, or dull my senses, I will remember even though I overeat in private, excess poundage is there for the world to see. I will take off pounds sensibly.*

If your weight loss support is lacking, TOPS is a great low cost alternative for support and weight loss education. With 10,000 chapters around the world, you're bound to have more than one near you.

LISTENER QUESTIONS

Q What should you do if your partner isn't supportive of your fat loss goals?

A Comfort in a relationship is a powerful thing. When one person in a relationship starts changing themselves, there is bound to be some push back from the other person in the relationship.

That push back may be your partner telling you that they were comfortable with the old, fatter you. You may have shared favorite, decadent foods. You may have watched more television on the couch together. Now that you're changing and leaving the comfortable life you are both accustomed to, they are now voicing that they don't like the new you, or worse sabotaging your weight loss endeavors. Here are some suggested choices to help remedy this situation:

Choice 1: You can go back to your old lifestyle. Grow fat and old together. That is what your partner is proposing.

Choice 2: Continue on your path and ignore their comments. Lead by example and maybe they will come around. You are going to have a body that gets better looking every day.

Find support elsewhere. Get your support from friends and coworkers or places like TOPS, Weight Watchers, or from online support forums, like our own fat2fitsupport.com. The people that frequent these places are in the same situation as you, trying to lose fat.

Choice 3: Bring them along with you. If you're going to work out, ask them to join you. Keep asking every time you work out. Unless they are completely hardened to the idea of being healthier, they may eventually relent.

Choice 4: Two can play at that game. Time to make them healthier, whether they want to or not. Try making small choices around the house that, when taken together, will make them healthier.

For example: Start buying healthier foods and skipping the less healthy choices. Eventually replace food with the healthiest alternatives. If they have a favorite recipe, change it to have less fat or get a replacement one that's just as tasty, but has less calories. Buy smaller plates. This is kind of a cheesy trick, but when people use smaller plates, they may still fill them up, but by virtue of their size they put less food on them. These are just a couple examples of some positive interferences that might make some small changes. Maybe they will lose a couple pounds and come over to your way of thinking.

> That push back may be your partner telling you that they were comfortable with the old, fatter you.

This is not a desirable situation. It is hard enough to lose weight with support. It makes it much harder when you don't have the support at home. Inevitably, it's your body and you are responsible for it. Do you want to live life to its fullest or just get by? Keep your goals in mind and no matter what your partner says or does, you can still be successful.

Chapter 46

"There are two primary choices in life: To accept conditions as they exist, or accept the responsibility for changing them." —*Denis Waitley*

FAT LOSS GADGETS

T HERE IS NO SUBSTITUTE FOR hard work when losing fat, but sometimes a weight loss gadget can make the process a little more enjoyable. Many of these electronic devices will strap to an arm or clip into a waistband. These devices can do everything from measuring your heart rate, monitor how many calories you burn and even track a run through GPS satellites. The key is to get the right one that will enhance your fat loss.

On one end of the fitness gadget spectrum is the simple pedometer. This little device tracks the number of steps a person takes. It clips on to your belt or waistband and an accelerometer of some kind clicks each time you move up and down while walking or running. When the pedometer knows how far your average step is, it will calculate the distance that you have moved.

Pedometers can be motivational if you use it to set distance goals for walks, runs, or even total daily activity. Pedometers are easy to find and can be quite inexpensive. At one point McDonald's was even giving them away with an adult "happy meal."

Top of the line pedometers with digital displays, electronic accelerometers, heart rate monitoring and GPS satellite tracking can be found at running stores and can cost several hundred dollars. After your activity, the data from the pedometer can be transferred into a computer where all of the recorded information can appear in charts, graphs, and even plotted on a satellite map.

At the other end of the spectrum are advanced devices called motion trainers. These devices have sensors that monitor and record things like your body temperature, your movement, and even your sleep cycles. When you connect the device to a computer, all of the recorded information will be available to browse through in simple and visual formats.

One of the most popular features of motion trainers is that they calculate how many calories you are burning minute by minute throughout the day. Based on your movements, it calculates your energy expenditure. When you also use the software to record what you eat, it will provide you with your daily caloric balance. On a daily basis, you will be able to monitor the "calories in versus calories out" balance. Motion trainer devices range from $100-$300. Two examples are Fitbit and Bodybugg.

For those that have a Smartphone, you have one of the greatest fitness gadgets ever invented right in your pocket already. There are numerous web sites and "apps" that are available for these phones. Some of these fitness apps can do all of the functions of a pedometer and a motion trainer. They can track your food and exercise, provide workout routines to follow, and can even turn the fat loss experience into a game, complete with lively characters and achievements that you can attain. Some of these Smartphone apps may be free or inexpensive.

One of the most popular features of motion trainers is that they calculate how many calories you are burning minute by minute throughout the day.

No device will make you lose weight. Losing weight is a matter of burning more calories than you consume on a regular basis. What these gadgets do is make that calorie counting and workout tracking much more enjoyable and easier to do. The assumption is that if it's easier, you'll do it more. Hence, you will have greater success. But don't feel like any device is required for you to lose weight. Hard work is all that is required.

THE CHALLENGES OF WEIGHT LOSS

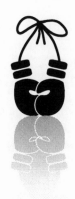

"An angry woman called 911 yesterday because McDonalds ran out of Chicken McNuggets. That is not cool. When you tie up the lines like that, 911 can't help people who are actually dying from eating Chicken McNuggets." —Jimmy Fallon

EMOTIONAL EATING

D EFINITION: EMOTIONAL EATING IS THE *practice of consuming large quantities of food, usually "comfort" or junk foods, in response to feelings instead of hunger.* Many people will find themselves in the drive-thru at a local hamburger place and not know how or why they ended up there. Chances are there was some external stimuli, probably negative and stress producing that led them there.

It could have been a bad day at work or perhaps someone or something really got on their nerves. It could have been the stress from the possibility of losing their job, or the partner that just won't get off their back. Even unhappiness about their current weight! Whatever it is, eating while emotional is disastrous for fat loss.

Here are the most common emotional eating triggers: Boredom, stress, fatigue, tension, depression, anger, anxiety, loneliness, negative self-worth, making excuses for eating, movies, sports events, advertisements for cheap food, skipping meals, or to "cure" some ailment like a headache.

If losing fat were as easy as eating less calories and exercising more, everyone would be thin. Who would choose to be fat? The truth is that 90% of weight loss happens above the shoulders. Your mind has to change in order to lose weight. Once that change happens, the body has no choice but to follow.

Those things that make us lose focus of our goals and produce stress in our lives can get the better of us. People want comfort from what ails them mentally, so they reach for the things that makes them feel better emotionally.

How do you stop emotional eating? If you feel the urge to eat, and you know it's not because you are hungry, do an alternate activity that will get your mind off of food and back to a good place. If the trigger is locational, or because of someone (spouse, mother-in-law), remove yourself from the situation and get into that alternate activity.

Here are some good alternative activities:

- Read a book or magazine
- Watch TV or a video
- Listen to music or a podcast
- Go for a walk or jog
- Take a bath
- Do deep breathing exercises
- Play solitaire
- Call a friend on the phone
- Do housework
- Mow the lawn or build a snowman
- Weed the garden
- Wash the car
- Write someone an e-mail or letter
- Meditate
- Or any other activity that you enjoy until the urge to eat passes

How about smoking? People can feel better when they smoke and feel some emotional release when lighting up. However, you are trading one bad habit for an even worse one. Probably not a good choice. The key is to replace the bad habit with a good one.

90% of weight loss happens above the shoulders.

If all these alternatives fail and you are going to eat to curb your emotions, try to limit the damage. If you know that you will eat when times are tough, prepare your home or office by removing high calorie foods that will derail your weight loss. Instead of keeping a pint of ice cream in the freezer for that time when you "need" it, fill your fridge, freezer and cupboards with healthy foods. Then even if you do overeat because of your emotions, you won't pack on pounds because of it. And don't make a shopping trip to the grocery store when you are feeling that urge to eat. Your cart will end up filled with Ho-Hos, Chocodiles, and Haagen-Dazs before you know it.

Finally, ask yourself one question: Will this food progress me toward my goal of losing fat? If not, then pass it up. Just a small pause before each meal, snack, or emotional eating attack, will go a long way in helping you achieve your goal of a healthy, fit body.

LISTENER QUESTIONS

Q I blew my diet for an entire week! I gained weight, and now feel guilty and depressed. What should I do?

A This topic was posted in our support group, and here are some suggestions from our listeners:

- Don't look back, start making the right choices now.
- Yesterday's meals don't matter. The only meals that matter are today's.
- The only thing under our control is the decision we make **right now**!
- Expect to get knocked down many times in your weight loss journey. You just have to stand back up, start again and persevere.
- One day or one week of bad eating will not kill you. That happens to everyone so enjoy it while it lasted, but critique why you did it, then forget it. Learning is the key.
- Did you have any success before last week? Do you weigh less today than a month ago (or six months ago?) If you do, you are still on a great course. Celebrate your accomplishments and build on them. Don't focus on one bad day or one bad week.

These are some great suggestions—simple and practical. The past is the past!

Chapter 48

"Though no one can go back and make a brand new start, anyone can start from now and make a brand new ending." —Author Unknown

FAT ENABLERS

A
N ENABLER IS SOMEONE WHO helps you do something. A "Fat Enabler," makes it very easy to put on weight and will support you in your obese and unhealthy lifestyle. An enabler can't make you overeat if you don't want to, but they can sure make it easier to do.

It is easy to think of extreme cases of people who are "Fat Enablers." There is the person who looks after a 1,200-pound bed-ridden person. They cook and provide all of the food for that person. They are clearly providing them with thousands of extra calories every single day.

Another example is a five-year-old child who weighs over 200 pounds. Clearly the parents are providing too much food on a regular basis and are responsible for making that child morbidly obese.

A bed-ridden, morbidly obese person and a very seriously overweight child have someone who is enabling them to be fat, but we all have people in our lives who enable us to be fat to some extent.

Before we trash "Fat Enablers" for making us fat, here are a few important facts:

1. You are responsible for what you eat and more importantly, how much you eat. So if you are hoping to blame your obesity on others, it doesn't hold much weight. Enablers make it easier to be fat and can sometimes outright encourage you, but you are the boss of you!

2. Someone who is an enabler isn't an evil person who wants to make you fat and unhealthy because that would make them happy. Generally, they want you to enjoy eating and your enjoyment from eating a tasty meal or snack or dessert is what makes them happy.

Here are 10 innocent examples of everyday fat-enabling examples.

- A spouse or roommate who buys junk food or snacks, so they are available in your home.
- A friendly coworker who always buys big party plates of appetizers for everyone to enjoy after work.
- A helpful spouse or roommate who buys take out on the way home all the time, so you don't have to cook.
- A loving spouse who has decided to show their love for you by making special desserts for you.
- Groups of friends who you only ever socialize with over dinner and drinks. The more you see your friends the fatter you seem to get.
- Many restaurants serve huge portions and most people will continue eating until their meal is entirely finished.
- The eager next-door-neighbor kid who is willing to do all of your outside chores for a few bucks.
- The family member who will go grocery shopping for you, so you can stay home and watch the big game.
- The partner who never gets on your case every time you need to buy larger clothing.
- Businesses that provide easy access to soda and junk food.

These examples do not force you to overeat and not exercise, they just make it much easier. It could be an escalator that makes it easier not to exercise. It could be a bus or a plane that now has wider seats and makes it more comfortable to be larger. There are many ways that people and things can enable you to be fat. So, how do you overcome people or things that enable you to be fat? Here is a simple three-point strategy. Be aware, challenge and then change.

1. **Be aware.** Is the situation encouraging you to be healthy or not? Simply ask yourself all the time, is what I am doing right now helping or hurting my health and fitness goals? How did I get in this situation?

2. **Challenge.** Make it known that this situation isn't helping you with your health and fitness goals. Sure, it makes you happy in the short term, but it makes all of your fat happy in the long term.

3. **Change.** Don't just say no, but provide alternatives. A person who is a fat enabler, is trying to please you. Allow them to do that, but suggest ways that would be healthier.

Every situation is different, but try to look at everything in your life and see if it is enabling you to be fat or fit.

LISTENER QUESTIONS

Q I am a very busy person, and most days I simply don't seem to be able to find the time to work out. What can I do so that I will actually start exercising more?

A There are millions of people who manage to regularly exercise who are just as busy as you, and just as tired when they get home from work. These successful people all have several things in common in their beliefs and how they stay motivated.

Here are three suggestions of how you can become more motivated to exercise:

1. You need to make yourself a priority. If you are extremely busy, you may need to schedule in a time that you will and must do your workouts. Your health is the most important thing to you, and you must believe it! Have you ever been too busy at work that you didn't go to the bathroom for 24 hours? Of course not. Just because your body can't scream out that you need exercise as loudly as you need to go to the bathroom, does not mean that it isn't as important. 10 years from now, you will still be in the same body, but your job may change. What should be your priority?

2. You need fitness goals. Just setting a goal to "get a workout in" does not cut it. What are you going to do? How long and at what intensity? Will it be an improvement on your last workout? Set daily goals the night before or first thing in the morning and make yourself accountable for their accomplishment. Those goals must also have a why attached to them. Who is going to exercise just for the sake of exercising when you are tired? Attach some powerful reasons.

3. If all else fails, get up earlier to exercise. Even if you are an extremely busy person with commitments and meetings that are always changing, early mornings are the one time when almost everyone can schedule a regular workout. The worst thing that could happen is that you will be tired for work instead of being tired for your exercise.

Chapter 49

"Keep steadily before you the fact that all true success depends at last upon yourself." —Theodore T. Hunger

PREGNANCY

ALL PREGNANT WOMEN WILL GAIN weight. It is part of the process. But how much weight should be gained?. In general if you are a healthy weight right now, you should gain between 25–37 pounds during your pregnancy. If you are underweight, from 28–40 pounds, or around three pounds more. If you are overweight, you should only gain between 15–25 pounds.

The weight that a mother gains comes from several sources. First and foremost, the baby. Newborns usually account for seven or eight pounds of the pregnancy weight. The placenta is about one or two pounds and amniotic fluid accounts for about two pounds. Through the process of delivering the baby, you will lose approximately 10 pounds.

Other weight will stick with you for a while. Your expanded uterus will still weigh an extra two pounds. It will get smaller as it contracts during the weeks and months following childbirth. A mother's lactating breasts will also weigh approximately two pounds more than normal. Fluids also accumulate in soft tissue and will add another four pounds. Then there are the things that you might not think about such as extra blood, about four pounds worth.

If you are carrying twins or triplets, you will obviously gain more weight, but your expected weight gain should not be double. It should be about 10 to 15 pounds more.

Before looking at problems associated with too much weight gain during pregnancy, there are risks when you don't gain enough weight. The main complication is low birth weight. These babies are categorized as SGA or small for gestational age. SGA means that they have been malnourished during pregnancy. Babies that are small for gestational age are also likely to be born prematurely.

The list of complications is much longer if you gain too much weight during pregnancy. Some of the problems will resolve with birth but others can cause problems for years to come. The list includes increased fatigue, leg pain, backaches, varicose veins, an increased risk of cesarean delivery, high blood pressure and gestational diabetes. If you have gained more weight than recommended during the beginning of your pregnancy, **do not** try to lose weight. It is never safe to lose weight during pregnancy. Instead, you want to **slow** your weight gain.

All pregnant women should eat a variety of foods to get all the nutrients you and your baby need. These are specific dietary suggestions to keep both baby and mother healthy:

+ **Choose lower fat items when eating out** such as broiled chicken breast sandwich with tomato and lettuce and a side salad and avoid fried foods such as French fries, mozzarella sticks, etc. that you might be craving.

+ **Avoid whole milk products.** It's recommended that pregnant woman drink milk, but choose skim, 1% or 2% to reduce the amount of calories and fat.

+ **Limit sweet or sugary drinks.** Sweetened drinks such as soft drinks, fruit punch, fruit drinks, iced tea, lemonade, or powdered drink mixes have plenty of empty calories. Choose water, club soda, or mineral water.

+ **Do not add salt to foods when cooking.** The salt will cause you to retain water and can increase blood pressure.

+ **Put away the donuts or muffins** and pick up a piece of fruit instead.

+ **Prepare meals using low-fat cooking methods.** Frying foods in oil or butter will increase the calories and fat of that meal. Baking, broiling, grilling, or boiling are healthier and lower fat methods of cooking.

+ **Moderate exercise can help you burn excess calories** while pregnant. Walking or swimming are both good choices for pregnant women.

There are several factors that will determine how fast a new mother can expect to lose the weight. First, if you gave birth through cesarean section, allow yourself ample time to recover from abdominal surgery. Assuming everything went well, after a few weeks of rest you can get started with working out again. Take it slow and don't over do it.

After delivery, there is extra fluid accumulated in the mother's body. These extra fluids can cause some discomfort, especially if localized in the extremities like the feet or legs. The fluids will be metabolized in the weeks following childbirth. It will almost seem miraculous as the fluid disappears and you recognize your feet again.

After your initial recovery period, losing the extra weight put on as part of your pregnancy is the same as any other weight. Any advice that we give you here in this book should apply to the new mother as well.

LISTENER QUESTIONS

Q I have lost a considerable amount of weight and now I have an unsightly bunch of skin that hangs around my middle/arms/buttocks/legs etc. My doctor has suggested cosmetic surgery to remove it, but is there anything that I can do without resorting to surgery?

A Skin is elastic, but there are many factors that will determine how elastic your skin may be.

Drinking more water improves the hydration of your skin much more than using moisturizers.

1. How long have you been overweight? The longer that you skin has been stretched out, the worse off you will be. After pregnancy, some women's skin will tighten back up fairly quickly, but after several pregnancies, it may never fully tighten back up again.

2. How large were you? This will determine the amount of stretching that has occurred. If you lost 30 pounds of fat, this should tighten up within a year. If you have lost hundreds of pounds of fat, the skin has not only stretched, but your body has grown more skin to cover yourself.

3. How old are you? As people age, their skin goes through many changes, and it takes longer for your body to heal.

4. Do you have good genetics? There is nothing that you can do about this. Some people naturally have better skin. Some women will show no signs of pregnancy only a few weeks after giving birth, some will show signs for the rest of their lives.

5. Do you eat, and have you been eating a nutritious diet and do you drink plenty of water? Your skin is your largest organ and eating healthy improves the overall health of all of your organs.

People think that special creams or lotions or oils that claim they can tighten skin or get rid of stretch marks or scars can help, but their effects are very minimal. It is true that moist skin is better than dry skin and many people use moisturizers. This may surprise many people, but there are now many studies that show that drinking more water improves the hydration of your skin much more than using moisturizers. The moisturizers affect mainly the outer layer of the skin, whereas drinking plenty of water hydrates from the inside out.

Skin does tighten up over time, but depending on all of those factors that we listed, it may never go back all of the way. There are limits to how much and how fast it can recover.

There are limits to how much and how fast your skin can recover.

This might seem obvious, but if you lose weight very fast, you will most likely get noticeable hanging and loose skin. If you lose it gradually, like we suggest, your skin might be able to keep up with your shrinking size.

The bottom line is that loose skin may or may not go away over time, but it is much easier to hide loose skin than bulging fat. And, while you may not like that loose skin, it will not affect your health in a negative way.

Chapter 50

"Don't measure a man's success by how high he climbs but how high he bounces when he hits bottom." —General George S. Patton

MEDICATIONS THAT MAKE YOU FAT

Disclaimer: *We are not doctors or health care professionals, and we are definitely not trying to give any advice as to what anyone should do with their medications. We are simply relating what the research shows, and if you want real advice about your specific situation and medication options, you need to talk to your doctor or pharmacist because they are the experts on this.*

MOST PEOPLE HAVE HEARD THAT there are quite a few prescription drugs on the market that have the potential side effect of making people gain weight. Jeff personally knows two people who suffered from mental illness to the extent that they were hospitalized. Within a year of being medicated with anti-psychotic drugs, they had both gained an extremely large amount of weight.

So how is this possible? Can a drug actually make you gain weight? We always promote on the show that it is just a matter of calories in versus calories out. Is it possible that by taking a certain medication, it could somehow overcome this basic law of energy?

Do medications just increase a person's appetite so much that they eat more, or can it have an impact on the speed of a person's metabolism, or is there something else that it could be?

According to the Therapeutic Research Center, a company which produces trade publications for doctors and pharmacists: *"Weight gain is a complex process involving both environmental and genetic factors. It is generally a result from an imbalance between energy intake and total energy expenditure. In addition to the many contributing factors to obesity, weight gain associated with drug therapy is becoming an increasing concern.*

"Many drugs have been reported to cause weight gain via different mechanisms. Drugs that commonly cause weight gain include mood stabilizers, antidepressants, anti-convulsants, corticosteroids, and certain diabetes medications."

These are the three ways that they suspect these drugs can make people gain weight:

1. **Your brain has many neurotransmitters that are associated with controlling your appetite.** If you are taking any drugs that work by changing the levels of histamine, dopamine or serotonin in your brain, they are shown to stimulate appetite and make you much more hungry.

2. **Certain antihistamines have sedative effects** and make you feel sluggish and lazy and just by decreasing your regular activity and not burning as many calories each day, this can lead people to gain weight.

3. **There are certain drugs that have the side effect of making people more thirsty**, and many of those people end up drinking more high-caloric drinks that makes them gain weight.

Here are more specifics about common drug classes that most people will end up using during their lifetimes.

1. Birth Control Pills

The most commonly used drugs thought to be associated with weight gain are birth control pills. Depending on which type you take, it may or may not be associated with weight gain. Oral contraceptives can cause a little weight gain by the retention of fluids and by increasing your appetite. They are not associated with any real significant chance of weight gain, and if you take low-dose products you shouldn't expect any.

There is one form of female birth control that shows a higher likelihood of weight gain though. This is the contraceptive injection that lasts three months and is commonly known as Depo Provera. This has been shown to increase appetite, but this doesn't mean that you have to give in to your increased appetite and overeat. Planning out your meals in advance is one of the best ways to deal with this.

2. Antidepressants

The next most commonly prescribed drugs are antidepressants. A quick Google search will turn up that more than 10% of Americans are on antidepressants.

There are a few antidepressants that are not associated with weight gain, but most seem to be. If they are a tricyclic antidepressants, or mono-amine oxidase inhibitors, you will generally put on more weight, the higher the dosage. What seems to happen is that people get an increase in appetite and cravings for carbohydrates and sweets.

The more common antidepressants are in the category called SSRI's or selective serotonin reuptake inhibitors. The good news is that they are more unlikely to cause you to gain weight. Your doctor or pharmacist will be able to tell you what you are taking.

The bottom line with antidepressants is that they increase cravings, but with goal setting and disciplined eating, it is not a guarantee that you will gain weight, any more than living next door to a pizza place is.

3. Mood Stabilizers

This category of drugs are to help stabilize a person's mood. These can be used to treat things such as bi-polar disorder or other types of mental illness. The most common drug that you might hear about is lithium. Lithium is one drug where it is fairly likely that you will gain weight. Studies show that after two years of treatment, the majority of people gain between 11 to 33 pounds of weight. It is associated with a dramatic increase in appetite and thirst in some people, but diet regulation and exercise has been shown to help in the studies.

4. Anti-Psychotics

Schizophrenia is a mental illness that is treated with anti-psychotic drugs. Those drugs are thought to cause dramatic weight gain by a combination of three things. First, they are sedating and make people sluggish and sleepy, they also slow down their metabolic rate, and finally they increase appetite. It isn't a good combination and these factors definitely can cause weight gain.

The two people the Jeff mentioned who gained a lot of weight, were taking anti-psychotics. 15 to 20 years after their bouts with mental illness, their weights are back down and they are healthy. This is one instance where we believe that you should take a medication even if it is likely that you will put on some weight. Deal with your mental health first, then you will have the rest of your life to live a healthy lifestyle and achieve your fat loss goals.

5. Hypoglycemics

The last type of drugs are hypoglycemics which are used to help control blood sugars in diabetes. Drugs known as insulin sensitizers, reduce insulin resistance in the liver and other cells and can be associated with fluid retention and the increased storage of fat.

Conclusion

The vast majority of medications that might cause the average person to gain weight, does not necessarily have to cause any weight gain. Here is the suggestion of what to do if you believe that weight gain is caused by medications. First in "doctor-ese":

"The first step in managing clinically relevant drug-induced weight gain is to consider switching to another agent in the same class associated with less weight gain if possible. If discontinuing the offending drug is not possible, behavioral modi-fication and dietary modification with increased physical activity should be considered."

Medications are just another challenge that can be overcome.

Translation: Number one, talk to your doctor about switching medications. Number two, set some fitness goals, watch what you eat and exercise. The bottom line is that medications can be a challenge for people. They can make losing fat or main-taining your weight harder, however they ultimately can't make you gain weight if you don't overeat. The law of calories in versus calories out still applies here. Some drugs can increase your desire to eat, but you ultimately are responsible for what goes in your mouth.

We all have challenges in our lives that makes it hard to be healthy and fit. Some people don't have a good support system in their lives, some have genetics that work against them, some have stressful jobs and fight daily to not use food for comfort. Medications are just another challenge that can be overcome.

Chapter 51

"In this age, which believes that there is a shortcut to everything, the greatest lesson to be learned is that the most difficult way is, in the long run, the easiest." —Henry Miller

FRAUDULENT FITNESS PRODUCTS

EFFORTLESS WEIGHT LOSS! LOSE 20 pounds this week! Drop a dress size overnight! Just six minutes a day! How can you tell which products are legitimate and which ones are fraudulent?

A small percentage of these products can help a consumer lose weight, but most are useless. If a fitness product or program sounds like it is promising too much for too little, it is. Any claims of easy, fast, hunger free weight loss are false. There has never been a true miracle diet or fitness program that has been developed. People want to believe there's a magic bullet. But there isn't one, despite all of the exaggerated product claims.

Fat loss comes from a calorie deficit along with exercise. That's it.

Fat loss comes from a calorie deficit along with exercise. That's it.

It is not just fitness gadgets that don't work. There are scores of overblown dieting and weight-loss systems. The Federal Trade Commission (FTC) found that over half of all weight-loss ads contained false or unsupported claims.

The agency says a red warning flag should be raised if a product promises:

- Weight loss of two pounds or more per week.
- Weight loss through blocking calorie or fat absorption.
- Weight loss attributed to wearing a product.
- Any program that promises extreme results for everybody.

So, if these products are fraudulent, and they contain unsupported claims according to the FTC, why are they selling them?

Many of these products are only sold for a short time. They advertise heavily, make their money, and then disappear. Many of these products make false advertising claims in order to make sales. Many of these product's manufacturers have lost class action lawsuits and received millions of dollars in fines. For many of these manufacturers, the fines and lawsuits are an expected expense of doing business. They continue to offer bogus products with false advertising claims, because they are still profitable in the end after all of the judgments and settlements.

One such individual, Kevin Trudeau, has been fined and sued for millions of dollars over a variety of products, including a weight-loss book, but is still ahead despite the legal issues. According to a FTC Press Release, Trudeau claims that the weight loss plan outlined in his book is easy, can be done at home, and readers can eat anything they want. When consumers buy the book, they find it describes a complex plan that requires intense dieting, daily injections of a prescribed drug that is not easily obtainable, and lifelong dietary restrictions.

You can't get the benefits of exercise unless you exercise.

In fact, in November 2007, Trudeau was found in contempt of the 2004 court order for making "patently false" claims in his weight loss book. The U.S. District Court Judge ruled that Trudeau "clearly misrepresents in his advertisements the difficulty of the diet described in his book, and by doing so, he has misled thousands of consumers."

Another example of fraudulent products are the electronic stimulation ab belts. The FTC charged three of the top selling ab stimulation products with making false claims. Here are some of the promises from these products:

- "Now you can get rock hard abs with no sweat"
- "Lose four inches in 30 days guaranteed"
- "30% more effective than normal exercise"
- "10 minutes = 600 sit-ups"

What words should set off alarms in your brain? How about the words "no sweat" or "guaranteed"? The FTC is charged with, among other things, protecting US consumers from unfair and deceptive acts or practices. When purchasing fitness equipment, the FTC advises consumers to:

- Ignore claims that an exercise machine or device can provide long-lasting, easy, "no-sweat" results in a short time. These claims are false: You can't get the benefits of exercise unless you exercise.

- Question claims that a product can burn fat off a particular part of the body — for example, the buttocks, hips or stomach. Achieving a major change in your appearance requires sensible eating and regular exercise that works the whole body.

- Read the ad's fine print. The advertised results may be based on more than just using a machine; they also may be based on restricting calories.

- Be skeptical of testimonials and before-and-after pictures from "satisfied" customers. Their experiences may not be typical. Just because one person had success with the equipment doesn't mean you will, too

- Do the calculations when you read statements like "three easy payments of ..." or "only $49.95 a month." The advertised cost may not include shipping and handling fees, sales tax, and delivery and set-up fees. Find out the details before you order.

On the topic of fitness equipment, the old adage "if it looks too good to be true, it probably is" is never more accurate. Weight loss will not come easy and won't come in a bottle you buy from the TV. It will, however, come from your hard work. Which of course corresponds with another old adage: "If it's worth doing, it's worth doing right."

LISTENER QUESTIONS

Q People are always telling me about some new diet program that I should try. Every diet that I hear about promises quick and easy weight loss, so how do you tell which ones are simply too good to be true?

A We get countless emails from listeners who ask us about diet programs and ask for our opinions on them. For most of the diets that we are asked about, it is very easy to find hundreds of testimonials on the Internet and several professional looking websites that support those diets. With so much misinformation and marketing hype out there, it is very easy for the average consumer to be swayed into trying out a bad or dangerous diet program.

Here are the three easiest ways to tell if a diet is too good to be true:

1. If a diet ever uses the terms "easy" and "fast weight loss," it is a scam. It is really that simple.

If it is not an outright lie, it will be a serious exaggeration. Many diets will say outrageous claims such as a "lose 1 pound per day without hunger" or "lose 10 pounds per week" etc. If it simply sounds too good to be true, it is.

There is never going to be a diet that will be fast, easy, and without any hunger. There are tens of thousands of diets being marketed today and none of them live up to those promises. To put it bluntly, every possible combination of factors has been tried in all of these diets. Any new "miracle diet" will simply be older diets repackaged.

> There is never going to be a diet that will be fast, easy, and without any hunger.

2. If a diet makes a claim that weight loss is based on one miracle factor that has recently been discovered, they are misinformed.

Weight loss is a combination of many factors such as quality and quantity of food you consume, the speed of your metabolism, the amount of exercise and activity that you do throughout the day etc. By manipulating these factors, it will account for 99.9% of your weight loss efforts. Diets that are based on single factors like hormones, your blood type, your body shape, supplements, vitamins, or even vitamin injections such as B12, are missing the boat.

3. Any diet program that does not want you to exercise is clearly not thinking about your health. Diets that claim that exercise isn't necessary do this for one of two reasons. First, they are trying to attract people who are looking for a quick and easy solution, and they know that more people will buy their diet if they can make it seem as easy as possible. Secondly, they may realize that because their diet is a starvation diet, people will not be physically capable of exercising while on their diet. Either way, long-term studies all show that regular exercise is one of the most important factors in all successful weight loss programs.

Chapter 52

"If you want to get somewhere you have to know where you want to go and how to get there. Then never, never, never give up." —Norman Vincent Peale

TOP WEIGHT LOSS PRODUCTS TO AVOID

L ATE NIGHT TELEVISION AND THE Internet are full of products that seem like they could help with weight loss, but the only thing they lighten is your wallet. During the course of the Fat 2 Fit Radio show, we have highlighted many products that will help you succeed in your fat loss goals. Some of the most beneficial products have been things like a large 12-month dry-erase board to set goals and mark your progress, a fitness ball, a body fat scale or even a small MP3 player or iPod to listen to your favorite music or podcast while exercising.

Here are some of the most useless weight loss products on the market today. These products only offer minimal benefit for a high financial price, or they have no plausible scientific mechanism for aiding in fat loss.

1. Fat Blocking Pills

These pills go by names such as Alli or Xenical. What they do is reduce the amount of fat that you can absorb by up to 25%. Remember that it's the overall number of calories that you eat that makes you gain or lose weight. "Fat makes you fat" was an '80s craze that was not backed up by science or any studies.

These products only offer minimal benefit for a high financial price, or they have no plausible scientific mechanism for aiding in fat loss.

Let's look at what you are actually saving by using these products. Consider a person with a 1500 calorie per day diet with 20% of those calories coming from fat. If you do the math, on one of these products you would not digest 76 calories derived from fat.

Where does that fat go? It goes right through you. Side effects include "oily discharge." That's hardly worth the money. Simply eat ⅓ cup less rice per day to get the same calorie savings without the financial costs and side effects!

2. Detox Kits

Your body gets rid of toxins in the liver. Humans have managed to survive for millions of years without any help removing toxins. Many people want to do a detox to start off a diet, but it is totally unnecessary. If you want to start off this year with yet another crash diet that harms your metabolism, go for it, but simply not eating any processed foods for a few days will have the same effect.

3. Electronic Ab Stimulation

These products were investigated by the Federal Trade Commission because of their false claims of fat loss and inch loss, and that they give users well defined abdominal muscles. These devices claim that they will give you the same or better benefit of conventional abdominal exercises such as sit-ups or crunches. None of these claims are true.

4. Whole Body Vibration Machines

These were all the rage in the '50s through the '70s. They didn't work then and they don't work now. The supposed theory of how they work has changed, but it is the same junk back again. Walking up a few flights of stairs will burn more calories and build more muscle than any of these machines ever could.

5. ROM Four-Minute Cross Trainer

This is an exercise device that sells for $14,615 mainly through magazine ads. It claims that you can get the body that you desire for only four minutes per day. If it sounds too good to be true, it is. You could pay for dozens of gym memberships for the same price.

6. Weight Loss Sauna Products

One sauna brand claims that you can "burn 900 calories in one hour" just sitting in the sauna. When you sit in a sauna, you lose a great deal of fluids through sweat. This might cause a sudden loss of a few pounds, but it is only fluid loss. When you re-hydrate your body, the weight will return. When your body is too hot or too cold, it attempts to regulate its temperature through shivering or sweating. This will burn a few more calories, but not to any significant level that would cause fat loss.

7. Diet Supplements

Claims that diet supplements make are not evaluated by a governing body. They are considered food, not drugs, and therefore are not monitored by the FDA.

Here's the rundown on diet supplements:

- They are not proven to work for any significant weight loss.
- They do not promote a healthy lifestyle.
- They can have serious interactions with prescription medications .
- The health risks are simply too great for no proven results. People often take too much and in combination with others and this can be simply dangerous.

8. Body Wraps

Herbal body wraps, widely promoted as a quick and easy way to lose fat and inches, are no longer just offered at spas. At-home versions abound, many of them sold over the Internet.

The claim: Just slather yourself with the mixture of herbs, minerals and other ingredients. Wrap yourself in terry-cloth strips and plastic wrap, and fat cells will move into your lymphatic system and out of your body forever. No study has shown that body wraps can reduce fat levels.

LISTENER QUESTIONS

Q I had weight loss surgery and it really messed up my metabolism. I ate so little when I was in the weight loss phase, that now that I'm in maintenance can barely eat anything without gaining weight. How do I fix my metabolism?

A This unfortunately is the reality for most people who undergo weight loss surgery. You may have a thinner body, but you suffer for the rest of your life from some of the side effects. Depending on the exact type of bypass, your body is now incapable of proper absorption of many things. This is why people who have undergone a gastric bypass need to be on vitamins and/or supplements for the rest of their lives.

In one of our shows, we had a lengthy interview with someone who had gastric bypass surgery a few years earlier. His weight had stabilized at 270 pounds and he claimed that he only ate 1100 calories per day. We are not sure how accurate his calorie counting is, but he has significantly messed up his metabolism by doing this. He is still well into the obese category, but to maintain his weight at 270 pounds, he still has to eat like somebody who weighs less than 100 pounds. That just doesn't seem fair!

People need to understand that in the quest to be thinner, you will never be able to enjoy food like you should be able to for the new size that you are. However, there are now probably hundreds of thousands of people who are in this situation, so here are our suggestions to try and get your metabolism going again.

> Each extra pound of muscle that you gain back, will allow you to eat an extra 30-50 calories more per day.

1.   **You need to eat more healthy unprocessed foods.** You also need to eat more often. Many people, who have had gastric bypass, eat unhealthy processed foods. Because they can't eat a lot at one time, they often eat things like crackers and snack foods. It is just much easier than preparing a tiny balanced meal. It is true that many are not eating a lot of calories, but you need to concentrate on eating non-processed foods. Get most of your carbohydrates from vegetables, and other healthy foods.

2.   **You may think that you cannot eat any more food without gaining weight.** That may be true if you don't also increase your exercise. By increasing your activity, it will speed up your metabolism. The way that you slow down your metabolism is by starving and not doing any exercise. The opposite will help.

3.   **You need to do resistance training.** Don't just casually lift two-pound dumbbells, do some moderate to heavy lifting. The amount of muscle that you have is the most important factor that determines how fast your metabolism is. A large percentage of your weight loss may have been from muscle loss.

   When you lower your calories too much, your body thinks that it is starving and it tries to conserve energy. Your body doesn't digest its own muscle because it needs the energy from the broken down muscle (you had plenty of fat for it to use), it is trying to offload the parts of the body that use the most energy. You need to try and gain that muscle back. Each extra pound of muscle that you gain back, will allow you to eat an extra 30-50 calories more per day.

4. **When you are doing resistance training, you need to also make sure that you are eating very healthy.** Putting on muscle is 30-40% what you do in the gym, and 60-70% proper nutrition. The most important thing is that you are eating lean protein with every single meal. The amino acids that come from protein are the building blocks of muscle.

These tips will work for anyone who has slowed their metabolism by dieting too fast or through weight loss surgery. It is just as simple as eating healthy, eating often, exercising regularly and doing resistance training to gain back lost muscle.

Chapter 53

"Your body is the baggage you must carry through life. The more excess the baggage, the shorter the trip." —*Arnold H. Glasgow*

HOMEOPATHIC WEIGHT LOSS PRODUCTS

I N 2007, THREE PERCENT OF Americans have used knowingly or unknowingly homeopathic remedies to fix a variety of ailments. One of the ailments that homeopathy claims to be effective against is obesity. A German doctor named Samuel Hanneman started homeopathy over 200 years ago. At this time in history, the germ theory of disease had not been discovered, and a common treatment for many diseases was blood-letting, where a person would be bled in order to get rid of "bad blood."

Homeopathy is the theory that a substance that makes you sick can cure you if it is diluted enough. So for example, if you have nausea, you would find something that would make you vomit. Then you would dilute it in water in a series of steps and then take the diluted form of it so that it isn't strong enough to make you ill.

> Mathematically and scientifically, in almost all homeopathic remedies, it is impossible that a single molecule or even atom of the active ingredient remains.

This goes against all common sense, but in homeopathic theory, the more dilute a medicine is, the stronger it is. Following this theory, if you had a glass of Kool-Aid, and poured it into a swimming pool, that swimming pool would now have a stronger solution of Kool-Aid in it. (This isn't a joke, this really is the current theory.)

Compared to medieval treatments of the day, homeopathy proved to be safe. The dilutions were so extreme that it was almost impossible that any of the original medicinal ingredients remained. Giving people "water as medicine" was safer than bleeding them.

Homeopathy proved to be very effective in curing ailments that would naturally get better on their own. The common cold gets better in seven to 10 days. If you use a homeopathic remedy to cure your cold, it will cure your cold in seven to 10 days ... The only benefit was that it didn't make things worse, like some of the medical treatments of the day would.

As science based medicine has progressed and changed over the last 200 years, homeopathy has not changed. Science has clearly proven that homeopathic remedies cannot work. In the early 19th century, it was proven that for these remedies to work, they would have to break the laws of chemistry and physics.

Mathematically and scientifically, in almost all homeopathic remedies, it is impossible that a single molecule or even atom of the active ingredient remains.

Currently, homeopathy proponents now concede that there is none of the active ingredients remaining in most remedies. Now the theory has slightly changed to include "water memory." Even if there is nothing left in the water, it will somehow remember the original "vibrations" of the substance that was in it before it was diluted. Remember the weaker the solution, the stronger the effectiveness of the solution.

So how do you tell if something is a supplement or a homeopathic remedy?

Most homeopathic products in North America look like any regular medicine that you would buy. If you read through the ingredients and the information, look for X's or C's. If you see numbers like 24X or 30C, it is a homeopathic product. That is often the only way that you can tell them from other products. It is more common in North America to see X's and in Europe to see C's.

There are no homeopathic weight loss remedies that will do anything to help with your weight loss.

These numbers refer to the amount of dilution of the active ingredients. Each time the number increases, the dilution is 10 times greater. So a regular product might be 30C or 30X and the extra strength product might be 40C or 40X.

So how dilute are homeopathic remedies? The allowable amount of arsenic in drinking water in the U.S. is one part per hundred billion. This is the same as 4C or 8X. That is a one with eight zeros after it.

Homeopathic remedies usually start at 24X or 12C, you have one part in 1×10 24th power—that has 24 zeros after it. This is the level where it is almost impossible to have any remaining atoms of the active ingredient. The strongest remedies are around 60X or 30C. That means that you will have one molecule in 1×10 60th power.

So which are the best homeopathic weight loss remedies? There are no homeopathic weight loss remedies that will do anything to help with your weight loss. Like all drugs and medicines, there may be a placebo effect. Some people will get a benefit from a product simply because they believe that it will help them.

If you happen to see homeopathic weight loss remedies mixed in with the supplements in a health food store, save your money and steer clear. If a salesperson or friend recommends that you try one of the products, politely say no and if they press, ask them about their understanding of how homeopathy works.

Most people can spot an obvious weight loss scam, but they can't spot homeopathic remedies when they get mixed in with real science based medicines. The only proven way for fat loss is by decreasing your calories and increasing your exercise.

WEIGHT LOSS IN THE REAL WORLD

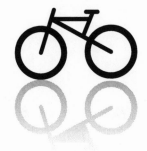

"Give me a stock clerk with a goal and I'll give you a man who will make history. Give me a man with no goals and I'll give you a stock clerk." —*J.C. Penney*

EATING HEALTHY ON A BUDGET

E ATING HEALTHY WITHOUT BREAKING THE bank is important for everyone. While there is an abundance of cheap food in the world and no one should go hungry, no one should go broke trying to eat healthy. Here are some tips to help you save some money:

1 Clip those coupons.

It's time-consuming and often they are for processed foods, but there are some good deals to be had. Just be choosy on the foods that you are saving money on.

The more you see a food product outside of the grocery store, the more it will cost you inside the grocery store.

2 Buy the less-expensive generic or store brands.

Store brands are often the same as the major label brands. We have been told by people on the inside of food packaging plants that the only difference in the major label and the generic label food is exactly that, the label. One listener wrote in and gave his account that they would put different labels on the same can of food depending on who the customer was. Typically the difference in price between the two is the amount of marketing that is put into the major label brand. The more you see a food product outside of the grocery store, the more it will cost you inside the grocery store.

3 Eggs and beans are great alternatives to meat.

Eggs get a bad rap because of people's belief that the cholesterol in eggs will raise their cholesterol. We recommend using one whole egg with six egg whites to get a cheap source of high quality protein. Beans, as well as having protein, are a great source of complex carbohydrates. Highly recommended.

4 Don't eat out.

Preparing your own meals is always cheaper and almost always healthier. You are not paying for the restaurant's rent, servers, cooks, electricity and the restaurant owner's profit. Take all that away and you will see that the $15 meal, could have cost you $6 at home. Plus, you are fully aware of the ingredients that are in the foods that you are eating. In one study, it was found that the number of calories that restaurants quote in their menus, if they do so, can be from 20% to 200% higher than stated. Good reason to stay home.

5 Buy lean meats in bulk, then divide up and freeze.

Meals should

be planned and

grocery lists

made before

heading out to

the grocery store.

Costco and Sam's Club are your friends when making large meat purchases. These companies buy in huge quantities and pass the savings on to the individual. In addition, many club chains, because they make money on memberships, cap the amount that you pay over their cost.

6 Don't go shopping when you are hungry.

Old wives are right about this one. Go shopping on a full stomach and you will resist more of those sweets that make you fat. Meals should be planned and grocery lists made before heading out to the grocery store.

7 Buy your produce at the farmer's market instead of the grocery store.

At the local farmer's market, Russ can buy a five-pound bag of oranges for $1. At the grocery store they are $1.29 a pound.

8 Don't buy sodas and other sugary drinks.

Drink water. Water is almost free and the money-saving benefits of drinking water are totally eclipsed by the positive health benefits.

Chapter 55

"Our greatest glory is not in ever falling,
but in rising every time we fall." —Confucius

SURVIVING A CRUISE OR AN ALL-INCLUSIVE RESORT

A VACATION FOR MANY PEOPLE IS a recipe for serious weight gain, especially when faced with unlimited decadent foods at buffets. It is possible, mindlessly eating and drinking while relaxing in the sun, to put on a pound or two per day.

A vacation is a time for relaxation, so one should enjoy it and not completely deny oneself. The key for most people is moderation. For many people, a realistic goal would be to maintain their current weight or only gain one or two pounds during their vacation.

> You have not "failed" the buffet if you didn't try one of everything at every meal.

The Fat 2 Fit Radio philosophy is to live the lifestyle of the thinner person that you want to become. That thinner person does vacation, and enjoys themselves (within reason), and maybe even gains a pound or two. When the vacation is over and they go back to their regular lifestyle and routine, any extra weight should disappear within a month without any effort.

Here are some specific tips to follow while on vacation:

- Take advantage of the gym. If you are on a cruise ship, there is most likely a walking/running track. If you normally exercise, don't stop because you are on vacation. Moderate exercise will help reduce any lingering stress and allow you to relax more.
- Sign up for classes like dance, fitness, yoga etc. that are offered. Some of them cost extra, but there are plenty that are included as part of the cruise or resort experience.
- Walk whenever you can and take the stairs instead of taking an elevator. There is no rush to get anywhere on vacation!
- Instead of picking sedentary excursions such as bus tours, choose the active

excursions such as kayaking, ATV or horseback riding.

- Eat breakfast, lunch and dinner in the dining room. Avoid the buffet at all costs if possible.
- If you must eat at the buffet, load up on fruit or veggies instead of pastas and breads. You'll eat a lot more food for a lot less calories.

Figure out which healthy strategies you use at home could be applied to your vacation.

- Decide before hand that you are only going to eat one plate at the buffet.
- Circle around the buffet first so you can plan what you are going to eat. Piling that plate high with every item in the buffet is a great way to overeat. Look at everything, then make your decision on what looks the best and the healthiest and just get those foods.
- Don't be afraid to customize your food at a "cooking station". There are often sandwich or pizza stations that will cook you exactly what you're looking for, no matter how decadent. Use that freedom to customize that food to be healthy.
- You have not "failed" the buffet if you didn't try one of everything at every meal. You will have multiple chances to try everything in the buffet at some time during your vacation.
- Alcoholic and non alcoholic drinks can have many calories in them. It is very easy to drink "slushy" or "fruity" drinks with syrup flavoring that can add literally thousands of calories and pounds of fat to your vacation. Even a can of soda or beer adds about 150 calories.

Final Points

- Don't try to be perfect—allow yourself a few free meals so that you don't feel deprived, but plan out before hand how many.
- You may not have a choice of foods, but you can always limit the quantity of the food that you consume.
- Figure out which healthy strategies you use at home that could be applied to your vacation with a little modification. For example, if you are used to having healthy snacks with you, plan ahead and take some pieces of fruit from the buffet for later in the day.
- If you keep a food journal, bring it along. This might be the best way to keep yourself from becoming blissfully unaware of what you are eating throughout the day.

Chapter 56

"When I was young I observed that nine out of ten things I did were failures, so I did ten times more work." —Bernard Shaw

CHILDHOOD OBESITY

OBESITY RATES FOR CHILDREN HAVE skyrocketed in the last 20 years. Here are some current statistics for the United States:

- It is estimated that 15% of all children are overweight, with another 15% at risk of becoming overweight.
- ⅔ of overweight kids will become overweight adults.
- Nearly 35% of children six to 19 are overweight. Half of those—nearly 11 million—are considered obese.
- Over the last 25 years, the obesity rate for young children has doubled and the obesity rate for teenagers has tripled.
- Diseases such as diabetes, high blood pressure and cirrhosis of the liver, which were previously only associated with adults, are now seen in children.
- The average lifespan of an obese child will be five years shorter than the lifespan of their parents.

How to know if your child is overweight

The way to tell if your child is considered overweight or obese is by the traditional Body Mass Index calculation method. Children's BMI is calculated a little differently than that of adults. It's the same BMI calculation, but compared among children of the same height and age. Like the adult BMI scale, it isn't perfect, but it is a starting point.

Causes of childhood obesity

Debate is ongoing as to the cause of the increasing obesity rates in children. Lawsuits against McDonald's and other fast food restaurants would have you believe that fast food is to blame. Another lawsuit blames Oreos because they contain trans fats.

Some of the other leading theories for the causes of childhood obesity are:

- Kids are less active—they watch too much TV and play a lot of video games.
- Fast food with high calories and high fat super-sized meals.
- All of the processed snack and lunch foods for children.
- Drinking soft drinks and sugary 'fruit' drinks.
- Buying in bulk, such as boxes of snacks from warehouse stores.
- Schools allow students to buy snacks and soft drinks from vending machines and don't always require physical education classes.
- Our culture is becoming a "culture of obesity."

It is safe to assume, that like adults, it's a combination of all of these factors and more that is making our future generations fat. Any single factor could cause a child's waistline to expand, but a combination of these is a recipe for a fat kid.

Who's to blame for childhood obesity?

A survey conducted by ACNielsen, found the following:

- 1% of parents blamed food manufacturers.
- 7% blamed advertising on TV, etc.
- 9% blamed the child.
- 10% blamed fast food companies.
- 67% of parents blamed themselves.

The majority of parents blame themselves for their child's weight problem.

With younger children, parents are the only ones that have control over all of the factors of obesity. Parents can help their children make healthy food choices, both at home and when eating fast food. Parents can limit TV watching and time spent playing video games, and can encourage more activity. Teaching our children to make healthier choices is ultimately the most important thing if we want them to avoid the negative health consequences of being overweight.

It is always best to be proactive early in life, and the earlier the better.

As teenagers, parents start to lose control over all of the food that they may be eating. For example, once they start to have their own money, they may start to eat more soda and candy on their own. When they head off to school, that nutritious lunch you lovingly prepared for them may end up in the trash, replaced by a burrito, chocolate chip cookie and chocolate milk.

What's the first step?

Before you try to have your child lose weight, your first goal should be to work with your child to stop gaining weight. This will be an easier first step for you and your child. After the weight gain has stopped, have your child maintain their weight for two to three months before you start any weight loss plan.

A good rule of thumb for child weight loss is one pound per month. You may see more weight loss depending the child's level of activity, but on average, one pound per month is a healthy weight loss goal. Remember that at the same time that your child might be losing weight, they are also growing. You do not want to stunt any potential growth by extremely limiting your child's calories.

Helping your child achieve their goals

Calories in versus calories out. The same philosophy that we recommend for adults in their fat loss is the recommendation for your child. With the recommended fat loss of one pound per month, the time-line for achieving your child's weight loss goal is a slow and steady one.

Analyze what your child is eating on a daily basis. Have a frank and open talk to your child about what they are eating during the day. You may pack their lunch each day, or think you know what is in the school cafeteria lunch, but you may find there are more opportunities for snacking than you think.

The next step is to look for areas where you can lower their calories. One major place to start is beverages. Chocolate milk, juices, sodas and flavored waters just add sugar and empty calories to their diet. Another great way to control their calories during the day is to pack a lunch for your child.

You should not punish a young child for eating. That will only cause negative associations with food and guilt about eating in the future.

Teenagers have very little impulse control. Food choices do not

> You should not punish a young child for eating. That will only cause negative associations with food and guilt about eating in the future.

often include any thought regarding nutrition or healthiness. A parent may have little control over what their teenager eats out of the home. One strategy to help a teenager is to help them with their motivation. Work with them to come up with many reasons why they want to do this. As well, set some goals and rewards. They must want to change for this to be successful.

Your child or teenager, while they may weigh more than is recommended, is still growing. If they grow a substantial amount—two inches in a year—their current weight may turn into their healthy weight.

Prevention

If your child is not overweight, there are a few things you do to help your child maintain a healthy weight.

- Avoid snacking.
- Reward with fruit instead of sweets.
- Give children low-fat snacks for their breaks and meals at school.
- Get children out of the house as much as possible by tying in computer games with physical activity games.
- Limit their use of computer games and watching TV.
- Make exercise a family activity, so that children learn that exercise is fun, not a chore.
- Get them involved in organized sports. Make sure that you find a sport that they like.
- Aim for a broad range of foods rather than excluding or severely restricting foods.
- Occasional burgers, sweets and chips are fine as long as they are balanced by other less fattening foods.
- Never outright ban a food—this will just make them want the banned food more (the kids who never get candy seem to buy it more when they can).
- You can't rely on a school's P.E. program to have a huge impact. The amount of hours in class is nothing compared to the rest of the week.

Ultimately, like your weight loss and maintenance of your ideal weight, it comes down to connecting the dots. What goes in the mouth has a direct relationship to what the body looks like and how it functions.

LISTENER QUESTIONS

Q How does alcohol affect weight loss?

A There are studies that show drinking one or two glasses of wine per day can improve long term heart health. However, alcoholic drinks do contain calories and are detrimental to people who are trying to lose weight.

Alcohol contains seven calories per gram. That is almost double compared to protein and carbohydrates, and only fat is higher at nine calories per gram. People who start drinking alcohol with their meals will start gaining weight if they keep eating the same amount as they always did. Extra calories regardless of the source can be converted to fat.

> While your body is getting rid of the alcohol that you have consumed, all fat loss stops.

Alcohol is treated differently in your body than the other macronutrients. When you have alcohol in your system, the alcohol is processed by your body first. Once all of the alcohol is gone from your system, then your body will start using carbohydrates and fat for energy. To put this another way, while your body is getting rid of the alcohol that you have consumed, all fat loss stops. No body fat will be used for energy while your liver is removing the alcohol from your system.

You may have heard that on some carbohydrate reduced diets, like the Atkins diet, they allow you to drink spirits because they do not have any carbohydrates. Those types of diets also acknowledge that spirits postpone any fat loss until the alcohol calories are used up.

Low-carb alcohol is no better for you. It will still slow down your fat-burning potential. The current "zero carb" campaign for vodka and whiskey is baloney and may encourage mindless consumption. It's like bragging that a candy bar is "cholesterol-free."

Here are some results of studies on alcohol:

1. In an *American Journal of Clinical Nutrition* study, there was evidence to suggest that consumption of alcohol leads to an increase in appetite over that of any other carbohydrate type drink.

2.   A study of healthy male volunteers observed that after drinking
     alcohol, the effects showed a significant decrease in testosterone
     and an increase in cortisol (a muscle destroying hormone) lasted up
     to 24 hours.

3.   Alcohol interferes with the metabolism of most vitamins, and with the
     absorption of many nutrients. Alcohol stimulates both urinary calcium
     and magnesium excretion. This means that you'll get less benefit from
     the "healthy" meal you may be consuming.

We are not recommending that people give up alcohol if you enjoy a drink
once in a while. Everything in moderation—live the perfect lifestyle 90% of the
time and don't worry about the other 10%.

Chapter 57

"There are no secrets to success: Don't waste time looking for them. Success is the result of perfection, hard work, learning from failure, loyalty to those for whom you work, and persistence." —General Colin Powell

"THE BIGGEST LOSER" PROS AND CONS

I N CASE YOU HAVEN'T HEARD of the popular television show "The Biggest Loser," it is simply a weight loss competition. People compete to lose the most amount of weight in the shortest amount of time for a cash prize. There are currently 25 different versions in production right now and these are seen in 90 different countries around the world.

Our philosophy on Fat 2 Fit Radio is for life-long weight loss success. It is 100% opposite of what viewers will see on "The Biggest Loser." We always say **not** to get caught up in focusing on losing big numbers every week, **not** to workout six to eight hours per day, and **not** to push yourself past what is medically safe for you and your current body. We conclude that if you do five percent of the effort that they do, you can easily have life-long weight loss success and fitness.

> We conclude that if you do five percent of the effort that they do, you can easily have life-long weight loss success and fitness.

Millions of people watch this television show, and there are some good points that viewers can get out of it. The most important thing is for people to be able to take the good from the show and ignore the bad points.

Pros

1. **It is entertaining.** The editing of the show paints compelling storylines in each episode, which makes it entertaining and emotional.

2. **They do have tidbits of information on nutrition and exercise that are helpful.** Over time, people can pick up many tips and tricks about nutrition and exercise just by paying attention to what the trainers and contestants say and do.

3. **It is motivational.** People see that it is never too late to make a huge

change in their life by losing weight and getting fit. It inspires many people to make a change in their lives.

4. **They acknowledge that weight loss is all about calories in versus calories out.** They eat lower calories to get in a caloric deficit and then do exercise to increase that caloric deficit to increase weight loss. Weight loss is all about hard work. They never get hung up on the latest supplement or type of berry or extract etc. to lose weight. They do it by eating less and exercising more.

Cons

1. **The fitness and exercise programs are extremely dangerous.** The show has contestants attempting intense activity, such as a one-mile race, on the very first day of training. A responsible, professional trainer coaching a person in poor cardiovascular shape and hundreds of pounds overweight, would **never, ever** put a person like this through an exhaustive workout on the first day. A person in this condition must move into a workout routine with a safe progression of intensity. People in this condition who attempt to model after the show are at a high risk of serious cardiac complications or even death.

2. **It is not possible for people in the real world to train like they do.** What the contestants do is clearly overtraining. Working out between six to eight hours per day does burn calories, but they are clearly on the thin edge of injury. Most people who attempt to do this amount of training will suffer a wide variety of overuse injuries within a few weeks. When people believe that they must exercise this much to lose weight, they usually give up on their weight loss goals when they become injured and can no longer exercise. The Internet is full of stories from people who have suffered this fate modeling after this show.

3. **The weight loss goals are unrealistic for people to achieve.** People have regularly lost 20 pounds in a week and people have been considered failures and voted off the show for only losing eight pounds in a week. Nobody can live up to those expectations. We all don't have millions of people watching us on television and personal trainers and masseuses and medical help and nutritionists etc. at our beck and call.

4. **How many people have given up on any weight loss because they have worked their butts off for a week and only lost three pounds?** If they have to work four or five times harder to live up to these elevated expectations, why should they even bother?

5. **This is a weight loss competition.** It doesn't matter if you lose fat, muscle, water or even bone. The goal is not to lose fat, only "weight."

Put another way, if you lose weight the healthy way, you will be unsuccessful on this show. If you only lose fat and keep all of your muscle, you are considered a failure here.

Here is a famous quote from season one winner Ryan Benson on his MySpace blog:

"I wanted to win so bad that the last ten days before the final weigh-in, I didn't eat one piece of solid food! I wore a rubber suit while jogging on the treadmill, and then spent a lot of time in the steam room. In the final 24 hours I probably dropped 10-13 pounds in just pure water weight. By the time of the final weigh in I was peeing blood.

"In the five days after the show was over I gained about 32 pounds. Not from eating, just from getting my system back to normal (mostly re hydrating myself). So in five days I was back up to 240—crazy!"

Kai Hibbard (season three) tells us about her final weight in on her MySpace blog:

"I dehydrated off 19 pounds in the last two weeks before the BIG weigh-in. I stopped eating solid food after eating only protein and asparagus (a diuretic) then I had two colonics and spent the night before the weigh-in, in and out of a sauna. There really was no 'diet' the day of the weigh-in, we weighed in as dehydrated as possible, on empty stomachs after two-hour workouts in the morning."

As with Benson, Hibbard's final week weight came flying back:

"I actually put on about 31 pounds in two weeks. After my body had a chance to stabilize I spent all last year hovering between 159 and 175, I fight everyday to find some stability."

This is **not** permanent weight loss and a lifestyle change! It is unfortunate that they are considered as weight loss role models for millions of people. The bottom line about the show is that it is entertainment. If people find it motivating and inspirational that is great, but realize that it is more Hollywood than reality.

In conclusion, "The Biggest Loser" is very similar to the show "Dancing With the Stars." The public's interest in dancing has skyrocketed, but what percentage of viewers can now dance like them?

LISTENER QUESTIONS

Q What do they do on "The Biggest Loser" to lose weight so quickly?

A On the television show "The Biggest Loser," they push people to their extreme limits for extraordinary "weight" loss. "The Biggest Loser" is a "weight loss" show and not a "fat loss" show. People do lose fat on the show, but they also lose weight through a loss of muscle, bone density, water etc.

We do not recommend that anyone attempt to follow these techniques that we will reveal here, but this is a very common question from our listeners.

In all cases, the contestants are eating below their Basal Metabolic Rates.

Weight loss is all about the calories in versus calories out equation. Each day the goal is to create a massive caloric deficit in order to lose "weight." They do this through eating very low calories and going through extremely long exercise sessions.

According to the nutritionist on "The Biggest Loser," contestants eat four cups of fruit and vegetables, mostly vegetables, lots of lean protein like turkey, chicken without skin, egg whites, red meat occasionally, and lots of dairy. A typical woman eats 1200 calories, the largest men (400+ pounds) may start at 2400. In all cases, the contestants are eating below their Basal Metabolic Rates. They also eat multiple small meals, usually three meals and two snacks per day.

Because their metabolisms quickly start to slow down by eating too little, they compensate through exercise. Contestants train between six to eight hours per day, and attempt to burn in the range of 3000 calories per day. The weight lifting, resistance training, chin-ups, etc. that you see on the show is mainly for the TV cameras. That is an extremely small portion of their training. Their main goal is to burn calories and they do this by doing extremely long sessions of cardiovascular exercise. They are spending time on ellipticals, stair climbers, bikes and treadmills at a moderate level of intensity to keep their large muscles moving hour after hour after hour.

Can a person in the real world do it?

The simple answer is no. First, they have daily medical supervision and receive all sorts of injections such as potassium and vitamins to keep them somewhat healthy as they are going through this starvation diet. Second, without all of their sports therapy support such as massages, physiotherapy, and other treatments, no untrained person could withstand those workouts without strains and overuse injuries. Third, without the psychological help, mentally people couldn't last more than a week or two under this much physical and mental stress.

> They will now have severely damaged metabolisms and when they can no longer spend hours every day to burn calories, they will quickly gain their weight back.

Is this a healthy way to lose weight?

No, this is a "weight loss" competition, not a "fat loss" competition. At the end of the competition, people will have to go back to their "real lives" and will not be able to train full time. They will now have severely damaged metabolisms and when they can no longer spend hours every day to burn calories, they will quickly gain their weight back. The contestants who seem to be able to keep their weight off after the competition, all seem to earn income from "The Biggest Loser" franchise.

Chapter 58

"Quality begins on the inside... and then works its way out." —*Bob Moawad*

INTERNET MARKETING FOR DIETS & WEIGHT LOSS PRODUCTS

T HERE IS A WHOLE WORLD of health and fitness related products and programs on the Internet that are being marketed to you. Just like in the real world, some of these products are total garbage and a waste of money, and some are pretty good and can deliver at least some of what they promise.

Affiliate marketing has become so popular and lucrative that it often creates a "distortion field" around promoted products.

When most people hear about a product, it is fairly easy to research that product through a variety of means. However, when you hear about a product on the Internet, and then search the Internet for reviews and more information, you may not be able to find factual information. For example, when researching a new diet program, you can spend hours researching and literally find hundreds of websites and blogs that rave about it. When you purchase the program, you may discover that it is only a three-page pamphlet!

With so much competition in the health and fitness category on the Internet, the products that people purchase are simply the ones that are the best marketed and advertised. That is true of the real world, but on the Internet there are many more "creative" forms of advertising.

The most popular form of marketing on the Internet is known as affiliate marketing. This type of marketing harvests the collective power of individuals to help promote products and services. One of the largest and most popular affiliate marketing programs on the Internet today is from Amazon.com. They pay out sales commissions for referring book buyers to their site. Almost anyone can join their affiliate program. Here is an example of how an individual would earn income from Amazon.com's affiliate program.

On a personal website, a person could list their five favorite books. They would add a link for each book that would go to the exact page on Amazon.com where that book could be purchased. If someone clicked on the link, and then purchased the book, Amazon would pay a sales commission to the referrer. In fact, in most cases, that sales commission is higher than what the author will earn for the sale of that book.

The vast majority of all fitness and diet products that you will find on the Internet are sold through this method. There are affiliate marketing companies, which bring sellers and promoters together. One of the biggest is Clickbank.com. This company runs affiliate programs for most of the health and fitness products sold on the Internet today.

At the time of this writing, its top 30 diet and health products all pay a commission rate of 75% of the full purchase price to the referrer. The top four affiliate programs are for diet programs. All of these diet programs pay more than $40 commission and claim that more than 90% of referrals will end up purchasing. One of these diet plans claims that their top affiliates sell over 100 products per day—that is $4000 per day in commissions!

The problem is that affiliate marketing has become so popular and lucrative that it often creates a "distortion field" around promoted products. So what are regular people doing when they find out you can make so much money promoting these products, many of which are pure garbage? Here are the six most common things:

1. **They are buying ads that appear on thousands of websites.** If it costs you $5 every time someone clicks on one of your ads, but you make $40, 90% of the time, how can you lose?

2. **People are creating websites for the purpose of putting affiliate links on their site.** The majority of fitness and diet websites today are there for the purpose of presenting ads/links to their readers. They have just enough content to look like a real website, but the website itself is only a few pages deep. They will often build their websites or even podcasts around the most lucrative products that they want to support.

3. **Why create one website, when you can create dozens full of affiliate links/ads?** The goal here is for people to accidentally discover these websites through Internet searches. These websites are full of very simple articles about diet and fitness. Mostly you will find "top five" or "top 10" lists of painfully obvious suggestions. The main goal of these sites is for you to see the ads, not read the articles.

4. **A common practice is for affiliate marketers to create fake product**

reviews to increase their sales. The sites that make the most money promoting products are all "comprehensive review" sites which will do fake reviews on dozens or hundreds of products. You may think that you are on a reputable site such as *Consumer Reports,* but you have fallen into an affiliate marketer's trap. The most commonly reviewed products are diet programs and diet supplements on these fake review sites.

5. **Many people create personal weight loss blogs and attribute their weight loss progress to certain products.** Many even say that they learned quite a lot from each of a variety of products and suggest that people try them out. This sort of "personal" affiliate marketing is unfortunately becoming quite common.

6. **The final and most insidious thing that people do is to create a really good website or podcast that gives out great advice.** The real goal of these sites is to collect email addresses. Many of these sites will only let you see certain pages when you provide an email address. Some sites will even offer some sort of free gift if you give them your email address. The most common way is to offer people a free monthly newsletter that they will receive through email.

   As they are growing their email lists, they will continue to provide decent content. At some point, those emails will begin to mention products and services that will pay commissions to the sender of the email. Affiliate companies are now even starting to pay a flat commission based on the size of the collected email list, even if nobody ends up purchasing a product. A company that has thousands of emails from people who are interested in diet and fitness, can sell those lists directly to marketers of health and fitness products. Most sites have disclaimers that they will not share or sell your email address, but unfortunately it isn't common practice to follow those disclaimers.

So this is the reality of weight loss and fitness products on the Internet right now. Just because something is being promoted through an affiliate program does not mean that it is garbage. It is possible that there are some diamonds in the rough.

So how do you know what is a good product on the Internet? You must use the knowledge that you have gained from reading this book, and your own common sense to evaluate these products. If they claim to have any sort of secret that they will tell you, or a revolutionary new discovery, or an easy and quick way to lose weight or get in shape, or in other words it sounds too good to be true, it is.

Chapter 59

"The best way to succeed in life is to act on the advice we give to others." —*Unknown*

HELPING OTHERS WITH YOUR NEW KNOWLEDGE OF HEALTH AND FITNESS

S THERE A LOVED ONE in your life whose health and well-being is at risk because of their obesity? Do you wish that you could share what you have learned about safe weight loss to them without seeming judgmental?

There are few discussions that you can have that are more awkward than a conversation with someone about their obesity. It's just uncomfortable to put yourself out there, especially when your input has not been asked for. There's fear of an argument or blowup, hurt feelings and dissolution of friendship and/or estrangement from family if it doesn't go right.

Despite these fears, expressing your concern may be the catalyst that might change their lifestyle for the better. Here are some suggestions to help you start that conversation.

- **Make sure you come from a place of concern.** Why are you raising the issue? Is it out of genuine love and caring?

- **Be absolutely certain you want to have the conversation.** Serious weight conversations like this are not the kind you want to have lightly. There are some heavy issues involved: self-worth, vanity, addiction, personal responsibility, stress levels, history, habit, family, and peer pressure are just a few. If you are willing to deal with them, great. If not, perhaps there's another way to help.

- **Consider approaching as a group.** When multiple friends or family members raise an issue with a loved one, it can show them the urgency of your message and make it clear that you are not the only one who sees the problem. However, before you sit down and talk, make sure that your group is all in agreement, with the same concerns and everyone comes across with the same positive solutions. You never want to gang up on someone who may already feel unhappy about themselves.

- **Don't wait until the last minute.** If you are truly concerned about someone's weight, the time to make your point isn't during their third bypass surgery. Though, when that loved one has a medical condition that is caused by their weight, that may be the opportune time to raise the subject.

- **Make sure you time it right.** Holidays and major life events cause enough stress as it is. Piling on, "Dad, I'm concerned about your growing belly fat" won't help. Pick a quiet time to start the conversation.

- **Don't assume they are unaware.** Odds are that someone seriously overweight is 100% aware of their situation. Also realizing that others are conscious of their weight can be severely embarrassing. They may have assumed that they've been hiding it well.

- **Ask the advice of a professional.** If you're feeling nervous or lost about where to begin, a doctor or fitness professional can give you some guidance.

- **Rehearse the conversation.** Rushing into important talks without a clear idea of what to say can leave everyone involved confused or angry. Think about your message. Frame it honestly and positively. Practice delivering it in the kindest tone possible. Anticipate responses. This isn't a debate, but being prepared can only help with the dialogue.

- **Don't be judgmental.** You are not the moral authority here. Casting aspersions or telling someone their behavior is a result of personality failure can make them defensive, angry, and/or sad.

- **Be honest.** Voice your concerns openly and kindly. Then, listen and ask and answer questions.

- **Use kind words.** Your choice of words could dictate how the talk is going to go. Avoid insulting language.

- **Use lots of personal references.** Relying on your own experiences is a great segue into talking about a loved one's. Try something like, "Dad, I've been getting a little gushy around the middle. I've been doing some research on losing weight. Have you read anything promising?"

- **Expect resistance.** "It's none of your business," "I'll never lose 100 pounds," or "I've tried dieting before, it doesn't work," are just a sample of the defensive responses you can expect. Don't take it as a personal attack. Accept it, make your points and keep moving.

- **Don't nag.** Nagging gets no one anywhere, ever.

- **You won't get instant results.** You have to understand that people change when they want to, not when you want them to. It's one thing to express concern, it's another to demand immediate change. You may be planting the seed that makes them start to think about their weight. Later on you might get a follow up question or invitation to coffee again, but only when they're ready.

- **Take one step at a time and be patient.** If your loved one is on the same page, offer assistance, and help them make small changes. Weight problems develop over an entire lifetime. You're not going to turn them around in day one. It will take time.

Made in the USA
Lexington, KY
15 June 2013